PRACTICAL DEMENTIA CAREGIVER GUIDE

EMPOWERING TIPS TO ELIMINATE BURNOUT, REDUCE STRESS AND STRENGTHEN RELATIONSHIPS

STEPHANE SUPPERVIELLE

ACKNOWLEDGEMENTS

To the Lord, the cornerstone of my life; to my wife, my source of boundless love and growth; to my children, for making me navigate the depths of love; to my family, for crafting a nurturing home, embodying unconditional love, symbolizing generosity, and instilling in me the desire to protect and empower; to my closest friends for supporting me; to my patients and their courageous caregivers, for helping me become whole; I dedicate this book to all of you, with heartfelt gratitude.

CONTENTS

INTRODUCTION

"Those with dementia are still people, and they still have stories, and they still have character, and they're all individuals, and they're all unique, and they just need to be interacted with on a human level."

– Carey Mulligan

When providing care for someone with dementia, you're taking on a significant challenge. Dementia, like Alzheimer's, brings about considerable difficulties. Recalling memories, thinking, communicating, and self-care become increasingly challenging. Mood swings and shifts in personality are also common. These changes deeply impact you as a caregiver. Whether managing daily tasks, making decisions, or simply offering support, you're dedicating a great deal of your life to another person. Your commitment and compassion shine amidst these struggles, illustrating the strong bond between you and your loved one. Handling the stress of caring for someone with dementia is not innate, and the changes in personality and behavior can leave you feeling lost.

Perhaps you are asking yourself:

- *What exactly is dementia?*
- *Where can I find information and support to navigate caregiving effectively?*
- *What should I expect in the days, months, or years to come?*
- *How can I best support my loved one?*
- *How do I handle challenging behaviors?*
- *What if I entrust my loved one with dementia to healthcare professionals, and something terrible happens to them?*
- *Am I making the right decisions?*
- *Why am I so emotionally drained and feel so alone?*
- *Is there a way to connect with my loved one despite their cognitive decline?*

Of course, you're right to ask these valid questions. And this probably isn't the first time you are looking for a proven way to deal with these problems. Or is it? Whatever the case, when you read this book to the end, you will understand dementia and its challenges at every stage. You'll learn to bond with your loved one who has dementia, even amidst mood swings and behavioral shifts. That is my mission and commitment to you.

Did you know that dementia currently affects over 55 million people worldwide, and this number is projected to *triple* by 2050, according to the World Health Organization? In the United States, like many other countries, caregivers for individuals with dementia bear a significant burden. The Alzheimer's Association notes that compared to all other caregivers, those caring for individuals with dementia experience "twice as many significant emotional, financial, and physical challenges." Meanwhile, an article in the *Dialogues in Clinical Neuroscience* journal highlighted how crucial caregivers are for people with dementia. Though challenging, it is essential for us to understand our loved one's reality and wishes. Our care truly matters – it keeps our loved ones well, and delays the need for institutional care.

You might think this is a big claim, but my experience supports this finding. I've seen firsthand the complexities of dementia behaviors, and I crafted this guide to assist you, families, and professional caregivers in navigating a way through them. In this guide, you'll get tools to communicate effectively and make informed decisions in the best interest of your loved one.

In my day-to-day life, I work alongside an interdisciplinary team of experts in managing the Behavioral and Psychological Symptoms of Dementia (BPSD). I am a board-certified music therapist and interact with dementia patients through music at a day center based in North America.

Music is a powerful tool to connect with people, even without verbal interactions. And music therapy refers to a credentialed professional's use of music to help their clients reach non-musical goals in the physical, psychosocial, cognitive, or spiritual domains. As a music therapist, I work within the humanistic framework through a resource-oriented approach. This means I see a person's strengths and focus on their well-being rather than on their dementia diagnosis. Trust is an essential component of this approach. A solid therapeutic alliance is necessary to uncover one's inner strengths and bring joy to their life through the power of music. And I am committed to sharing this approach with you.

In this book, I will guide you to start seeing your loved one with dementia through the same lens I do. Together, we will learn how to tap into your loved one's strengths, celebrate their well-being, and create moments of joy. We will see how to convey genuine empathy, respect, and tolerance rather than judgment. Some key ingredients of this approach are openness and honesty (the congruence principle), and seeking informed consent whenever possible, especially in important decisions that may significantly impact your loved one's life.

Although it is not always easy to do with dementia (or any other condition where one's perception of reality is altered), we will discuss the importance of communicating and making decisions based on what you know or think your loved one would have wanted if they could make informed decisions; even if they contradict your own beliefs.

We will explore strategies and solutions for what you can do as a caregiver, and help you find support for what you cannot do. The objective is to help you have the best possible relationship with yourself, your loved one with dementia, the healthcare professionals you interact with, your family, friends, colleagues, and society. Ultimately, this will help you get the best quality of life. And, believe it or not, you *can* experience joy, peace, and happiness amidst suffering.

The ***Practical Dementia Caregiver Guide*** takes a broad, holistic approach to dementia. It applies to settings varying from personal homes to long-term care facilities such as retirement communities, assisted living facilities, memory care, group homes, and nursing homes. Each chapter begins with a fictitious story featuring "Lovely", a woman diagnosed with dementia, and her adult children devoted to her care. Following each narrative, we will delve into practical insights that hold significance for caregivers. Once you've journeyed through this book, you will be able to:

- Understand dementia and act based on this understanding;
- Discover the roles and benefits of over twenty healthcare professionals in the dementia realm and how to partner with them;
- Know where to find professional help according to your financial resources;
- Foster understanding by placing yourself in your loved one's shoes, creating a positive atmosphere during interactions;
- Utilize a practical blueprint, knowing what you can control, what to do, and what to avoid;
- Learn how to engage your loved one's attention using easy methods and activities, even in times of challenging behaviors;
- Prioritize self-care, ensuring your well-being to offer genuine comfort and support;
- Manage stress effectively, thus preserving your resilience and guarding against burnout;
- Recognize the signs that specific services or accommodations are needed;
- Navigate family relationships throughout the diverse stages of dementia;

- Uncover the transformative power of peer groups, tapping into a wealth of shared experience;

The ***Practical Dementia Caregiver Guide*** isn't just a resource; it's my way of standing by your side. It is built upon the belief that well-trained people provide the best care. It isn't just a book; it's a lifeline. It equips you with tools to enhance interactions and quality of life for your loved one and for yourself.

The journey may seem daunting. You may feel overwhelmed by the myriad information out there and might not know where to turn. But don't worry, I did the legwork, so you don't have to. All the information you could possibly need is included within these pages. And if you want to jump to a specific topic at any time, please feel free to use the handy "Quick Reference Guide" at the end of this book.

As we embark on this journey together, remember that the challenges are real, but so are the rewards. Your commitment isn't overlooked; it's celebrated; and your dedication is an inspiration.

So, are you ready to make a difference? Then, let's get empowered!

CHAPTER 1
FUNDAMENTALS TO UNDERSTAND WHAT DEMENTIA IS

"C*aregiving often calls us to lean into love we didn't know possible."*
– Tia Walker

Lovely was a hardworking little girl who lived with her mother, Sophie, in a small cottage in the countryside. Her father had passed away when she was young, so it was just the two of them against the world. Lovely and her mother were best friends and did almost everything together.

Lovely's childhood was a simple but happy one. She would spend her days playing in the fields with her mom or helping her with the house chores. Her mother was a dedicated seamstress, but also had an interest in livestock and music. Lovely learned how to make clothes and assorted dresses. As she grew up, she took on more responsibilities in her mother's shop and tending to her mother's livestock.

Lovely also developed an interest in music and enrolled to sing in the choir at her local church. Her mother would sit in the congregations every Sunday to watch her sing and dance. Lovely felt safe and content living with her mom. However, one day, Lovely's mom fell ill with a severe illness; despite the doctors' best efforts, Lovely's mother passed away, leaving her alone.

Lovely was only seven when it happened, so she was devastated by the loss of her mom. She struggled to come to terms with her new life, and constantly lived in fear of abandonment, even after being taken in by her only surviving relative. She had everything she could ask for while growing up in her uncle's home, but still held on to the feelings of loss that would not heal… until she met Jack.

Lovely had always dreamt of finding true love, and she did when she met Jack, with whom she fell in love at first sight. She couldn't help but feel all that fear going away with her newfound love. Lovely and Jack spent all their time together, going on romantic dates, exploring nature, and visiting the big city. They quickly fell deeply in love, and Jack proposed. Lovely accepted, without hesitation. They were married in a beautiful ceremony and Lovely felt safe all over again. After a few years of marriage, the couple had two children, named John and Jennifer. The four of them lived happily together for a long time.

However, that happiness came to an end with the death of Jack many years later. Lovely was sixty-seven years old when this happened, and the familiar feeling of loneliness returned. Though devastated, she decided to live in her home alone and was content with her decision. But her children, who were grown, didn't let her go through it alone. They visited her as often as possible and showed her love and support. They knew their mother needed them now more than ever.

During one of the visits, Jennifer was shocked to find the house messy. She also discovered other disturbing matters, like her mother hadn't paid her taxes in eighteen months, which was most unusual. To make matters worse, Lovely often repeated the same questions. Jennifer realized her mother was forgetful about many things, and compensated for this by writing them down. Doing this helped her say the right things during conversations, even if she was secretly confused.

Jennifer also noticed her mother no longer did certain things she loved doing not so long ago. For instance, Lovely once loved exploring nature in any weather. But now, she mostly kept to herself in her room. No one noticed these changes except Jennifer. But every time she expressed her concerns to her mother, Lovely always denied that anything was wrong. She couldn't bring herself to tell Jennifer she was slowly losing her mind.

Eventually, Lovely agreed to visit her General Practitioner, who referred her to a neurologist for cognitive tests. Subsequently, the assessment ruled out other possible causes and confirmed dementia was the root cause for Lovely's symptoms. A few months later, after further testing and consultations with various specialists, the doctor diagnosed Lovely with Alzheimer's disease; dementia officially became part of Lovely's, and her family's, life.

On one fateful day, Jennifer walked into her mother's room to find a distressing sight. Lovely had fallen from her bed, and was lying there in a state of profound weakness and confusion. She couldn't move or utter a single word. So Jennifer immediately rushed her to the hospital.

Lovely didn't know what was happening during the first few days there. She was in a strange place, and nothing seemed familiar; even the people walking in and out of the room were strangers. But actually, Jennifer had told her where she was multiple times.

After much discussion and consideration, John and Jennifer decided the best thing for their mother would be to move her in with Jennifer, who lived in a spacious house with a large garden. They wanted to create a comfortable and familiar environment for their mom; a place where she could feel safe and loved.

The day before Lovely was discharged from the hospital, John went to their mother's house to collect her belongings. He and his sister planned to decorate Lovely's new room with familiar items that would remind her of their old home. John carefully packed Lovely's favorite clothes, her treasured photo albums, and her beloved collection of porcelain figurines. He also took her favorite armchair, which she had spent many hours sitting in, knitting, and singing her favorite songs.

When he arrived at Jennifer's house, he began decorating Lovely's new room. He arranged her clothes in the wardrobe and put her photo albums on the bookshelf. He placed her armchair in the corner of the room, next to the window. He knew this would be her favorite spot in the house, where she could sit and watch the birds in the garden. As John and Jennifer stood back to admire John's work, they felt a sense of satisfaction. They knew their mother would be comfortable in her new home, which was all that mattered. They hugged each other tightly, knowing they had done their best for their beloved mother.

The next day, Lovely was discharged from the hospital, and her children took her to Jennifer's house. She soon figured out that some of her belongings were missing from the room, and wrongly thought someone had stolen them while she was sick. However, Jennifer explained to her mother that there have been some changes and they would be living together now.

Lovely didn't like this new development. She had vowed independence after her husband died, and preferred to live in her own home. She didn't want to burden anyone. But as her life continued in this different environment, people would visit her and leave, and memories would appear and then vanish. She became baffled by the slightest changes in her routines. And unfortunately, Lovely soon couldn't tell the difference between reality and memories of people from her past.

Lovely's cognitive decline caused her to interpret ordinary sounds as louder than they were, and she felt agitated by the continuous movement of people in the dining room. Sometimes, she remembered their names. Most times, she did not. Usually, she forgot they had visited the previous week, and would constantly scold them for abandoning her. Friends and family grew more uncertain how to interact with Lovely as she continually echoed the same question, "Why have you left me here? I want to go home."

Lovely's story depicts some of the most common changes in people suffering from early to moderate stages of dementia, and more specifically, Alzheimer's disease. Individuals differ in their reactions to this condition, of course. So, one person's symptoms may vary from another's depending on their age, type of dementia, area of the brain affected, lifestyle, physical health, environment, etc.

WHAT IS DEMENTIA?

The brain is a highly complex organ with many pathways called neurons that allow us to do the fantastic things we do. Because of the brain's complexity, disorders can arise from even minor miscommunications between cells. Dementia is a blanket term that describes different chemical and structural imbalances which progress through and permanently damage the brain.

Dementia is not classified as a mental disorder, but as a neurocognitive disorder because it primarily affects cognitive functions. Thus, dementia is *not* an illness but the result of an underlying neurological condition called, "neurodegeneration." This is described as the slow and evolving loss of brain cell function until the cell eventually dies. It may also result from a disruption in the communication between nerve cell synapses rather than cellular death.

REGIONS OF THE BRAIN WHICH CAN BE AFFECTED BY DEMENTIA

Because dementia results from neurodegeneration, it can take many forms, depending on which area of the brain is affected.

Below are the larger regions of the brain that dementia could affect and their functions:

- The frontal lobes are the most prominent in the human brain and are responsible for voluntary movement, expressive language, logic, and reasoning. As a result, damage to the brain's frontal lobe causes problems with planning, decision-making, judgment, and impulse control.
- The temporal lobes are the second most prominent region located behind the ears. They are mostly related to the processing of auditory information and memory encoding. Overall, damage to the temporal lobe affects one's memory, hearing, and comprehension.

Within the temporal lobe, the limbic system is a collection of structures responsible for emotion, sexual desire, learning, and memory. Damage to the limbic system can throw the hormonal system off balance. The ability to sense hunger or satiety (feeling overly and uncomfortably full) is impaired when this happens, and mood swings become more common.

Within the limbic system, the hippocampus aids in learning new information. Hippocampal damage can lead to short-term memory loss, cognitive impairment, depression, and epilepsy.

- The parietal lobe is one of the brain's primary lobes, positioned in the top rear of the skull. It interprets sensory information from the outside world, primarily touch, taste, and temperature. Damage to the parietal lobe may result in sensory impairment, like accurately perceiving pressure, temperature, pain, and touch. Tying shoe laces may become impossible, for instance.
- The occipital lobe analyzes information from the eyes and translates it into the world as we see it. When the occipital lobe is impaired, vision difficulties, such as blindness or blind spots, as well as visual distortions and inattention, might occur.
- The cerebellum controls voluntary movements, including eye movements, balance, posture, walking, and motor coordination. Thus, damage to this area may cause difficulty dressing, inability to evaluate distances, loss of balance, and more frequent falls.

The following illustration will give a more detailed account of the functional areas of the brain and what they do.

DEMENTIA AND FUNCTIONAL REGIONS OF THE BRAIN

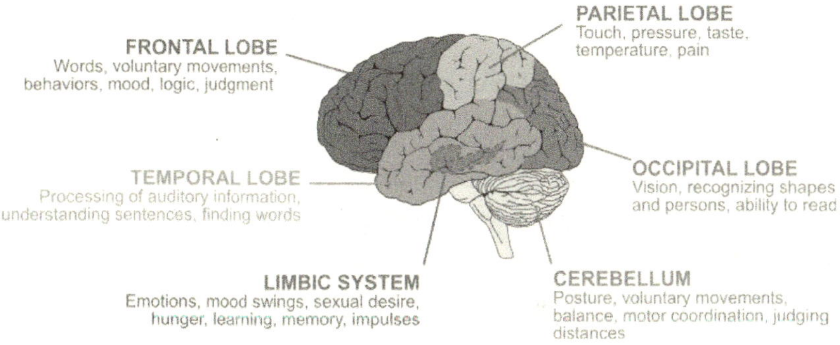

Now that you've learned about how dementia affects various brain regions, let's take a look at some of the ways you might notice those effects playing out in your loved one's life.

SYMPTOMS OF DEMENTIA

Symptoms that may appear *before* a dementia diagnosis are as follows:

- Forgetting recent conversations
- Forgetting names of close acquaintances or family members
- Memory lapses for recent events or facts
- Difficulty in finding the right words, often accompanied by frequent pauses
- Trouble concentrating or maintaining focus
- Difficulty in following and engaging in conversations
- Feeling disoriented about time and place
- Struggles with planning, organization, and problem-solving
- Challenges with coordination and motor functions

Cognitive impairment alone does not necessarily indicate dementia, and can result from many factors beyond dementia (e.g. substance abuse, mental health conditions, medications, infections, nutritional deficiencies, etc.). Therefore, consulting a physician for a formal assessment of the underlying cause of the cognitive impairment will be necessary.

NORMAL AGING VERSUS COGNITIVE IMPAIRMENT

Normal aging is a natural process that occurs over time and is characterized by gradual changes in physical, mental, and emotional well-being. While aging is a universal experience, the speed and severity of these changes can vary from person to person. Understanding the normal aging process can help individuals prepare for and manage these changes as they occur.

Physical changes are a common aspect of normal aging. Our bodies undergo muscle mass, flexibility, and coordination changes as we age. These can lead to a decreased ability to perform physical activities, an increased risk of falls, and a decline in overall physical health. Although undesirable, these changes are considered normal and sometimes called "pure aging."

As we grow older, recalling or processing new information may become more challenging. It is perfectly normal to feel concerned about shifts in our mental abilities. But mental changes are also a part of getting older, and the following signs are more often due to normal aging:

- Forgetting the name of an acquaintance you don't see often
- Forgetting details of a conversation or event from years ago
- Worrying about memory, but friends and relatives are not
- Having occasional difficulty finding words
- Occasionally forgetting things and events

However, if your loved one exhibits the following symptoms, you should suspect something more serious:

- Failing to identify the names of family members
- Forgetting about recent events or conversations
- Denying or overlooking memory problems that are obvious to family and friends

- Pausing often or substituting words frequently when speaking
- Having more recurrent memory lapses. If it happens to get to this point, it is critical to consult a specialist. Start with your loved one's general practitioner.
- Some other symptoms of cognitive impairment that justify consulting a doctor would be:
- Getting lost in familiar places
- Repeatedly asking the same questions
- Becoming more disoriented about time, people, and places
- Not taking care of oneself—eating poorly, failing to bathe, or driving dangerously
- Having trouble following recipes or directions

It's important to highlight that within the spectrum between typical aging and dementia lies a condition called Mild Cognitive Impairment (MCI). MCI is characterized by mild cognitive changes that don't significantly disrupt daily life, thereby distinguishing it from more severe conditions like Alzheimer's disease and related dementias.

THE SHOCK OF THE DIAGNOSIS

Being diagnosed with dementia significantly affects your loved one and you, as the caregiver. For your loved one with dementia, it could seem like their world is crumbling down around them, while you could be left extremely overwhelmed and discouraged. It's an experience that can be deeply distressing.

Take Lovely, for example; she had difficulty accepting her new condition and lashed out at virtually everyone. She had never expected that she would struggle with dementia and thought her life was over. This sentiment reflects the fear, disbelief, and dismay your loved one could experience after being diagnosed with dementia.

It is important to realize, however, that the time it takes to get a proper diagnosis for dementia varies and depends on several factors, such as the type of dementia, the individual's symptoms, and the availability of resources. A comprehensive evaluation for dementia can typically take several weeks to a few months and even up to a year or more. They usually include multiple medical and neurological exams, laboratory tests, and imaging studies. Obtaining a definitive diagnosis can also involve repeated assessments to track changes in the individual's symptoms and cognitive functioning.

Some of the typical tests and procedures used to diagnose dementia are:

1. **Memory and thinking tests**: Used to check how well the person remembers things, thinks and solves problems. Specialists may conduct **special cognitive tests** (if needed) to understand specific cognitive problems.
2. **Medical history checks**: The doctor talks with the person and reviews their health history, medications, and family history.
3. **Physical exams**: A thorough check-up to look for any physical issues affecting thinking.
4. **Blood tests**: To help find any health issues causing cognitive problems.
5. **Brain scans - MRI (Magnetic Resonance Imaging) or CT (Computed Tomography):** Special pictures of the brain to see its structure and check for any problems.
6. **PET (Positron Emission Tomography) scans:** Show how the brain uses glucose to help identify dementia patterns.

We can't stop at the diagnosis though. Next, we need to explore the different *forms* of dementia because your loved one's treatment will depend on the type of dementia they are suffering from.

FOUR PRINCIPAL FORMS OF DEMENTIA

Contrary to popular belief, dementia is multifaceted. According to Alzheimer's Disease International, there are more than 100 forms of dementia. However, we will look at the four most common types.

. . .

Alzheimer's Disease

Alzheimer's disease has become the most widespread form of neurodegeneration, comprising about two-thirds of all dementia diagnoses. Alzheimer's disease affects around 5.8 million people in the United States, according to current estimates.

It is a gradual condition caused by the abnormal accumulation of tau proteins and beta-amyloids in and between nerve cells. Generally, the anomaly starts in the brain's hippocampus, which, as discussed earlier, is strongly associated with memory.

The primary risk factor for Alzheimer's disease is age; most cases occur in people aged sixty-five or older. Another risk factor is gender, as Alzheimer's occurs twice more often in women than men. A common misconception regarding this is that women live longer than men, but recent research does not support this assumption. Instead, it correlates more to a robust immune response toward Alzheimer's disease in women than in men. At this point, you may wonder, "Wouldn't a stronger immune response help the body combat Alzheimer's, like any other disease, and thereby, protect women better than men?" Well, recent findings suggest that amyloid– a component of Alzheimer's disease – might be deposited as a defense against brain infections. And, as part of their enhanced immune systems, women may consequently produce more amyloid plaques than men, which would actually place them at a higher risk of developing Alzheimer's. So, it seems that more isn't always better. This complex interplay between gender, the immune system, and Alzheimer's disease is still an active area of research.

The typical symptoms of Alzheimer's disease are short-term memory loss, inability to learn new skills, and language disorders, leading to misspeaking or misunderstanding.

Although Alzheimer's disease, like all types of dementia, is currently incurable, chemical and psychosocial treatments are available to alleviate behavioral symptoms and delay the rate of cognitive decline.

Individuals may respond differently to medications, and dosages may vary depending on several factors, including overall health, but Cholinesterase inhibitors like Donepezil, Galantamine, and Rivastigmine generally help improve communication between nerve cells in the brain during the beginning stages; while Memantine regulates brain functions like learning and memory in moderate to severe stages*.

*Always seek advice from qualified healthcare professionals on any treatments.

Vascular Dementia

Vascular dementia ranks the second most common type of neurodegenerative disease, accounting for approximately one in every five cases. It can coexist with Alzheimer's disease or other types of dementia, which specialists refer to as "mixed dementia."

Vascular dementia encompasses challenges in reasoning, planning, judgment, memory, and other cognitive functions, stemming from brain damage due to inadequate blood supply.

Conditions such as strokes can block arteries in the brain, yet not all strokes lead to the development of vascular dementia. Similarly, other disorders affecting blood vessels and circulation can also deprive the brain of vital oxygen and nutrients, contributing to the onset of dementia. After the age of sixty-five, one's risk of contracting vascular dementia doubles every five years.

Below are some of the symptoms related to vascular dementia:

- Difficulty thinking
- Difficulty processing visual information in complex or cluttered environments

The condition of the brain's blood vessels significantly influences the likelihood of developing vascular dementia. Adhering to specific steps to ensure heart health may potentially reduce the risk of vascular dementia:

- Maintain healthy blood pressure levels
- Manage or prevent diabetes
- Cease smoking habits

- Monitor and regulate cholesterol levels

Lewy Body Dementia

Another common, though sometimes misdiagnosed, type of dementia is Lewy body dementia. This is the third most prevalent type of dementia, accounting for up to 10% of all cases in the US. The reason Lewy body dementia is misdiagnosed is because it could be involved in nearly one-third of all dementia cases when combined with other types of dementia.

Lewy body dementia is due to the formation of clumps of alpha-synuclein proteins known as Lewy bodies in the brain. Symptoms of Lewy body dementia (LBD) often present as a fusion of Parkinson's and Alzheimer's symptoms. These may include rhythmic shaking of hands and limbs, slowed movement, rigid muscles, alterations in speech patterns, difficulties in planning or problem-solving, memory loss, and challenges in completing routine tasks. Additional distinguishing factors of LBD encompass delusional thinking, visual hallucinations, difficulties in maintaining wakefulness, impairments in speech and swallowing, alongside loss of smell or taste.

Individuals diagnosed with Lewy body dementia may encounter intervals of lucidity interspersed with episodes of confusion and irrational thoughts. Lewy body dementia, as with other forms of dementia, cannot be prevented or cured. However, some symptoms may respond favorably to treatment, at least for a while.

Frontotemporal Dementia

While Alzheimer's disease attacks the hippocampus, frontotemporal dementia targets the frontal lobes. Neuronal loss in this area results in mood, behavior, and communication changes. Unlike other forms of dementia, one of the risk factors involved with this condition is genetics.

Frontotemporal dementia is ranked the fourth most common type of dementia, with a prevalence of about 3% of all dementia cases. It is, however, the most common type of dementia affecting people between ages forty-five and sixty-four.

Its symptoms are as follows:

- Obsessive behaviors
- Impaired judgment
- Apathy

The behavioral variant of frontotemporal dementia (bvFTD) is associated with the frontal lobe. It results in symptoms such as difficulty in planning and sequencing, changes in behaviors and personality, disinhibition (impulsive, unrestrained, and unconcerned about consequences), and socially inappropriate behaviors related to sex, food, alcohol, emotions, and actions.

The other form of frontotemporal dementia is primary progressive aphasia (PPA). This form is associated with the brain's temporal lobes, and its symptoms include severe language and comprehension impairments and difficulty swallowing. The famous American actor Bruce Willis was diagnosed with PPA.

Unfortunately, drugs commonly used in other types of dementia are not recommended for frontotemporal dementia because they can worsen the symptoms. On top of that, there is currently no medical treatment to slow the neurodegeneration progression rate. However, doctors may prescribe antipsychotics to decrease hallucinations or aggressive behaviors.

Although all dementia types have fundamental differences, they do share some common characteristics, and knowing them is essential to help you care for your loved one with dementia. The similarities are as follows:

- All types of dementia affect at least two regions of the brain
- Their symptoms gradually worsen over time
- Up until this day, they are all incurable
- They are all eventually fatal

In the late stages, when neurodegeneration affects almost the entire brain, the symptoms are very similar, regardless of the type of dementia. However, early-stage symptoms are quite different, which highlights the importance of knowing more about the various stages of dementia. So, this is what we will discuss next.

STAGES OF DEMENTIA

With a fundamental knowledge of the stages of dementia, you can help provide the care and support your loved one needs as their condition evolves.

There are different stage models used to track the progression of dementia. Each one focuses on evaluating the level of cognitive impairment. We'll look at two of the most essential, the 3-stage and 7-stage models. Note that some of the symptoms described in different stages may often co-occur, making the boundaries between stages tricky to gauge.

The 3-Stage Model

Early Stage

In the early stage of Alzheimer's disease, the person is still autonomous in their day-to-day life, but will start having memory lapses, and may struggle to make plans or decisions. They may also begin to misplace objects and need help finding things, or have trouble pronouncing words. In this phase, they might still be able to hide what's happening and compensate for these losses, for instance, by writing down important details.

The early stages of vascular dementia are similar to those of Alzheimer's, except for the main symptoms, which are difficulty planning and making decisions, rather than memory lapses. People may also experience mood swings, slow thought processes, and physical problems like vision or speech deficits.

In Lewy body dementia, early signs may be attention and awareness impairments, and visual (sometimes auditory) hallucinations.

In the early stages of the behavioral type of frontotemporal dementia (bvFTD), people may start displaying selfishness, apathy, disinhibition, overeating, impulsivity, aggression, and disregard for typical social rules. People in the early stages of primary progressive aphasia (PPA), the second type of frontotemporal dementia, may have difficulty recalling names, understanding conversations, and pronouncing words.

Middle (Moderate) Stage

In the moderate or middle stage, symptoms align across all types of dementia. Although some distinct features remain, such as motor degeneration in Lewy body dementia or social misconduct in frontotemporal dementia, the early-stage symptoms inevitably worsen. As a result, patients may be confused about concepts like time and place. They may also struggle to remember the names and birthdays of close relatives or significant anniversaries.

In the middle stage, your loved one with dementia may need help with some daily tasks, which healthcare professionals call "activities of daily living" (ADLs). In addition, they may start developing infections, such as urinary tract infection and pneumonia.You might also observe changes in their personality, triggering emotions of “ambiguous loss” for you as a caregiver*.

*I will explain the concept of ambiguous loss in more detail in the next chapter.

Late (Severe) Stage

The severe or late stage of dementia is characterized by physical decline and further cognitive deterioration, such as the inability to speak and disorientation regarding people, places, time, and situations. The symptoms of this stage are similar across all types of dementia, and constant care is required. Your loved one may no longer be able to swallow or walk. Risks of infections such as urinary tract infection and pneumonia, a common cause of death for people with dementia, also increase.

The 7-Stage Model (Reisberg et al., 1982)

The 7-stage global deterioration scale (GDS) model is pertinent to Alzheimer's, focusing on more granular memory loss and cognitive decline levels.

In stage 1, your loved one with dementia has no memory loss or impairment.

Stage 2 looks like the level of cognitive decline associated with normal aging, with a few memory losses, especially in unfamiliar situations.

In stage 3, however, close relatives notice unusual memory loss or language-related issues.

Stage 4 often matches with confident and formal diagnoses of Alzheimer's disease from a healthcare professional. Symptoms include:

- Short-term memory loss.
- Forgetfulness about familiar or personal details.
- Difficulty thinking and solving simple arithmetic problems.

Stage 5 is characterized by required assistance for certain activities of daily living. In this stage, your loved one with dementia is so disoriented that it becomes dangerous to let them live alone.

In stage 6, memory loss worsens, and your loved one with dementia may no longer recognize family members.

In stage 7, your loved one with dementia can no longer communicate, and physical systems deteriorate until they completely shut down.

To determine the stage of dementia, healthcare professionals often utilize the Clinical Dementia Rating scale (CDR). This assessment tool employs a five-point scale across six cognitive domains: memory, judgment, orientation and problem solving, home and hobbies, community affairs involvement, and personal care. While primarily utilized for Alzheimer's disease, the CDR scale can also assist in identifying stages of Lewy body dementia and other dementia types.

The length of time your loved one spends in each stage of dementia is primarily determined by the type of dementia they have and their specific medical condition. The average life expectancy for an individual diagnosed with Alzheimer's disease ranges from eight to ten years. However, some can live more than twenty years. The average life expectancy of people with vascular dementia is five years after diagnosis, while that of those with Lewy body dementia is six to twelve years after diagnosis. For people with frontotemporal dementia, the average life expectancy is six to eight years after diagnosis.

With our understanding of dementia deepened, we turn the corner into Chapter 2, which shifts the focus to your incredible role as a caregiver. On an airplane, when the cabin gets depressurized, parents are told to put on their oxygen masks first before helping their children. It's kind of the same for caregivers. You need to make sure you're okay so you can be there for your loved one. You need to have enough air to help. That air is filled with love, kindness, energy, and dedication in caregiving. Think of the upcoming strategies depicted in Chapter 2 as your oxygen, empowering you to make sound decisions and provide tender, compassionate care. This journey isn't just demanding; it's an opportunity for growth and connection that begins with you. Nurturing your well-being is the foundation for effective caregiving.

CHAPTER 2
A THRIVING SELF-CARE PLAN FOR CAREGIVERS

> "*It is not the load that breaks you down. It's the way you carry it.*"
> – Lou Holtz

With every day that passed, Jennifer grew to hate the word "fine" even more. Having witnessed her mother's early stages of dementia first-hand, in the beginning, she too believed Lovely would be "fine." After all, she had managed well after her husband's passing. However, the gradual shift from child to parent in decision-making overwhelmed Jennifer. Days turned into weeks, weeks turned into months, and Lovely continued to reside with Jennifer. The erosion of her mother's autonomy in daily activities added another layer of challenge, weighing heavily on Jennifer's heart as she navigated this complex care journey.

Fortunately, family and friends were very present at the beginning. They often called and visited to check on Jennifer and her mother. And although they didn't partake in Lovely's care as much as Jennifer did, their support went a long way in encouraging her.

Regrettably, the warmth from family and friends started to fade.

Their visits became less frequent, and they ceased bringing Lovely's favorite dishes. Additionally, they spent less time with Lovely, diminishing Jennifer's desperately needed respite time. They stopped visiting because they had noticed Lovely's declining cognitive abilities and didn't know how (nor want) to deal with them.

Lately, Jennifer's poor eating habits had caused her to gain weight. Her once impeccable hygiene was lacking as she got used to eating microwavable meals, fast food, and snacks with high sugar content. Worse yet, Jennifer's physical appearance was diminishing, and her mood swings became more frequent.

To top it all off, her mother's mental health was deteriorating rapidly. It got to the point where Lovely could no longer dress herself, or even remember her way to the toilet. She also refused to wear a pad, which forced Jennifer to clean the house and do laundry constantly to avoid her home from smelling awful. It was becoming too much to handle.

Dementia enormously impacts family and friends, and living with a person with dementia is often very stressful. Jennifer's case was no exception; especially as her mother's dementia progressed into the moderate and severe stages, accompanied by personality and behavioral changes.

Observing the gradual decline of a loved one from an independent to a dependent individual can be a harrowing experience. Not to mention, the demands on the time and emotions of the caregivers can be draining. Several family members have shared their dementia caregiving experiences with me. Many often felt sad, discouraged, and alone. Others occasionally felt angry and guilty about the situation.

Emotional stress is normal and understandable in caring for a loved one with a chronic condition; however, you must keep hope. Identifying the boundaries of your role as a caregiver can help you do just that. You won't be let down once you discover the tools to manage stress through a thriving self-care plan.

UNDERSTANDING THE KEY ROLE OF A CAREGIVER

Caregiving should not be characterized only by its negative attributes. Many caregivers have reported experiencing heightened feelings of love and affection for their loved ones with dementia as they embark on their caregiving path. This sense of connection often deepens as caregivers feel profound gratitude for the sacrifices their loved ones have made for them, especially when caring for parents or spouses.

Yes, caregiving is full of challenges. But for many caregivers, it allows them to broaden their life experiences and offers opportunities for personal growth and self-discovery. As a caregiver, you may find yourself acquiring new skills and gaining a better understanding of your capabilities. It's important to acknowledge that many caregivers step into this role with no prior training (and often with no warning) when their loved one is diagnosed with dementia and can no longer manage their daily activities independently.

You might have embraced this new role from a positive angle, believing you can show up for your loved one with dementia when they need it most. On the other hand, you might have felt apprehensive about becoming a caregiver. You may have experienced self-doubt, hesitation, and worry. This wide range of feelings is completely natural; every caregiver eventually experiences at least some of them.

Regardless of what you feel, try not to judge yourself.

Dementia often changes a person's behavior, making daily activities a significant challenge. So, even if you are an enthusiastic caregiver, you may still feel helpless as you try to understand your loved one's unusual behaviors. In this role, it's essential to recognize the importance of caregiving as a shared responsibility. Everyone, including caregivers, deserves care and support.

Here are some key areas to consider:

- **Healthcare management:** Caregivers play a vital role in managing their loved one's healthcare, including medication administration, monitoring their physical and mental health, and communicating changes to healthcare professionals. Medication adherence is crucial to prevent illness or complications arising from memory problems.

- **Assisting with daily activities and personal care:** Caregivers provide practical support, such as bathing, dressing, grooming, and meal preparation, to ensure their loved one's well-being.
- **Housekeeping:** Maintaining a safe and comfortable living environment is crucial for those with dementia. It includes checking the safety and security of the home, cleaning, and supervising to prevent accidents, like leaving the stove on or wandering.
- **Providing emotional support:** Emotional support is essential for preserving the dignity, comfort, and well-being of the person with dementia. Caregivers can offer support through physical touch, reassurance, and active listening.
- **Managing finances:** Caregivers often manage their loved one's finances, ensuring their financial security and stability. It includes organizing documents, budgeting, and paying bills.
- **Planning and organizing activities and appointments:** Effective planning and organization help meet the needs of the person with dementia while also reducing stress for the caregiver. Creating schedules, using time management apps, and encouraging social engagement are essential.
- **Mediator:** Caregivers may need to mediate conflicts and mollify situations where dementia-related symptoms lead to challenging behaviors like agitation or aggression. In these situations, you will have to pick up the role as mediator, helping to manage the situation and reduce stress for your loved one and their social network (siblings, children, close friends, extended family, etc.). Understanding your loved one with dementia's perspective is crucial to this role. Acknowledging their needs and anxieties will help them feel heard and validated.

- **De-escalation:** Outbursts and agitation are common symptoms of dementia. So, when your loved one becomes uncharacteristically aggressive, you must be able to identify their behavior as part of their condition and apply your training to calm them down.
- **Companionship:** Isolation and depression can occur when your loved one can no longer interact with their immediate surroundings as they used to. You know your loved one's social limitations and should carry out the appropriate emotional support and companionship response.

To summarize, taking on the role of a dementia caregiver is both challenging and compassionate. The responsibilities encompass a wide range of tasks that hold immense importance. Acknowledging the significance of your role is of the utmost importance.

REALIZING YOU ARE A DEMENTIA CAREGIVER

Simply put, a dementia caregiver is one who provides quality care to a person with dementia by tending to their physical, emotional, psychosocial, spiritual, financial, and legal needs. For instance, if you regularly take your spouse, parent, or friend with dementia to the doctor, buy their groceries, support or advocate for them, then *you* are a dementia caregiver. And it is necessary to recognize that what you do in your caring role is essential. What you do matters; you must own your role and the responsibility to do it well. You may need to remind yourself right now, "I am a caregiver, and I do the caregiving here." Step up. Own it, care for your loved one, but remember to care for yourself as well.

ACCEPTING THE DEMENTIA DIAGNOSIS OF A LOVED ONE

Sometimes, friends or family members, including those caring for a loved one with dementia, can be in denial and have difficulty accepting the dementia diagnosis; perhaps because of the possible changes it will bring to their own lifestyle and routines. At other times, the person with dementia might be the one in denial. Still other times, it's their partner because they're terrified of the unknown changes that will inevitably come to their relationship. However, as the condition progresses, those around the person with dementia will eventually accept the reality of the diagnosis.

What does this mean for you as a caregiver? You may have to explain to family, friends, and even your loved one with dementia that it is natural to be concerned when such drastic changes appear because you have no control over them. But accepting these adjustments will help you provide proper care and support.

The five stages of grief, as defined by Elizabeth Kübler-Ross in 1997, can further help us understand why so many caregivers struggle to accept the dementia diagnosis of a loved one:

1. **Denial**: In the initial stage of grief, caregivers employ denial as a mechanism to manage the weight of the news. During this phase, life can feel meaningless and overwhelmingly burdensome. The shock and disbelief surrounding the diagnosis and its implications for the affected individual are prevalent during this stage.
2. **Anger** is part of the healing process and may be directed at anyone, including your loved one with dementia. It could result from the fact that they can no longer do the things they once could. It's important to recognize that anger is a natural facet of the grieving journey and typically wanes over time when it is openly expressed. Nonetheless, the more deeply you feel anger, the more it will dissolve, and the sooner you will heal.
3. **Bargaining:** Before accepting reality, you will want to do anything to save your loved one with dementia. You may promise them you'll be kinder if they regain their memory, or vow to God to do something in return for sparing them. After all, we want things to return to normal and for our loved ones to be restored.

4. **Depression:** After bargaining, your attention shifts to the present moment. Then, you may feel empty and experience a deeper level of grief than anticipated. Depression crushes your spirit and impairs your ability to cope, and suddenly, you just seem to stop caring about everything. This depressive phase seems to last indefinitely. However, it does not align with the chronic psychiatric condition outlined in the DSM5 (Diagnostic and Statistical Manual of Mental Disorders, Fifth Edition), the reference book for mental health professionals. Instead, it is an appropriate reaction to unexpectedly sad news.
5. **Acceptance** is frequently misconstrued as being "all right" or "OK" with what has happened, but this is wrong. Most people never feel "OK" or "all right" after hearing their loved one has been diagnosed with dementia. In this stage of grief, the goal is to embrace the reality that your loved one is now cognitively deteriorating, and to understand that this new reality is the permanent reality.

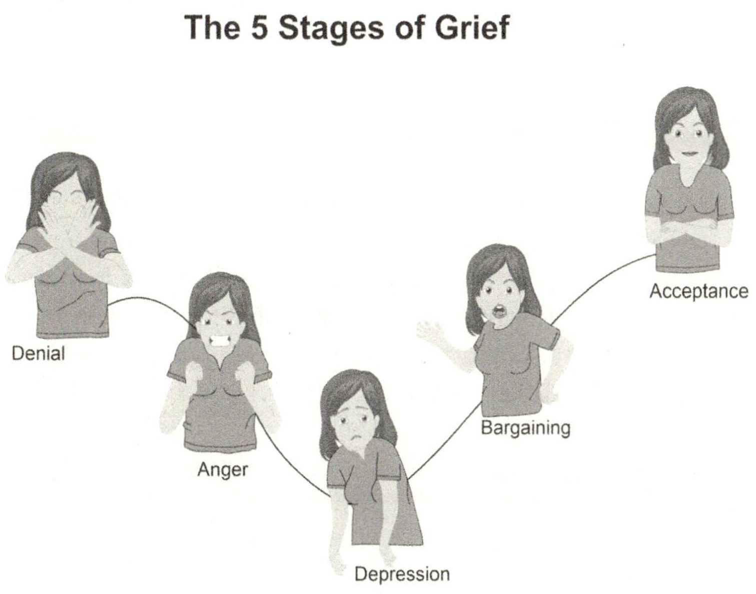

You may never fully agree with this truth, and you may not like it, but you ultimately need to accept it. As difficult as it may be, you have to come to terms with it since this is the new norm you must learn to live with from now on. You may find yourself striving to live in a world where your loved one may see you, but not recognize you. And acceptance of this fact may be even more challenging for you as a caregiver who interacts with them often. The reason I say this is because you might experience something I briefly touched on in the last chapter. It's a concept called "ambiguous loss."

AMBIGUOUS LOSS

Ambiguous loss is a situation that can arise from various circumstances, including physical loss, where there is uncertainty about the return of the person, and no confirmation of their passing. Ambiguous loss can also stem from mental changes, such as those associated with dementia, where there's no guarantee of a return to their previous cognitive state. For instance, you mourn the absence of a loved one who is physically present but profoundly altered due to dementia.

If your loved one has been diagnosed with dementia, you face a unique challenge. They are *here*, yet you've lost a significant portion of your previous connection to them. Recognizing that the person you were familiar with may undergo changes in behavior holds great significance, while concerns about their safety and the uncertainty of their experience only add to your worries.

In coming to terms with this new reality, understanding 'ambiguous loss' becomes essential. This term, employed by clinicians and researchers, encapsulates the journey you are undergoing—a journey that can be profoundly distressing. Ambiguous loss can be a traumatic experience for caregivers, potentially leading to burnout. Fortunately, there are strategies that exist to beat burnout, and you will discover them a little later in this chapter.

MAKING YOUR CAREGIVER JOURNEY MEANINGFUL

Caregivers travel a unique and winding road that is sometimes hard to understand when caring for a loved one. While caring for a loved one in need can bring great joy, the journey forward presents some unique concerns and issues.

However, there are ways for you as a dementia caregiver to find happiness as you tread this path. One way is to articulate the positive aspects of your role.

- **Why are you a caregiver?** This question is fundamental, especially if you had complicated relationships with your loved one before the onset of dementia.
- **Are you a caregiver out of love, duty, fear, or guilt?** Perhaps you want to set an example for your children, feel you have no choice, or offer caregiving as a community service.

Whatever your reason, you are here; you did not abandon your loved one with dementia. Find a clear, positive purpose and ways to value what you do, then write them down in a diary. Journalling will help you organize your thoughts, step back, and find clarity. Amid the uncertainty and hardships, find encouragement by returning to this precious "why."

STRESS ON DEMENTIA CAREGIVERS

The burden a caregiver must bear includes several components: financial effects, social isolation, "sandwich generation" difficulties (caring for children and parents simultaneously), and impacts on personal health. Needless to say, stress levels in dementia caregivers can rise rapidly, and burnout can easily occur without solid support networks. This can threaten the physical, mental, and emotional health of both the caregiver and their loved one with dementia.

Stress and depression are connected. While they are distinct conditions, chronic or severe stress can significantly increase the risk of developing depression. In addition, stress is often considered a contributing factor in the onset and exacerbation of depressive symptoms. Caregivers with negative opinions about their ability to cope and those who feel trapped in their responsibilities are more prone to develop depression symptoms. Additionally, they may experience a more significant burden when caregiving intensity increases, especially if they receive fewer benefits for their invaluable services.

By understanding stress and developing coping skills, you will equip yourself to face many challenges. Let's take a closer look.

What exactly is stress?

Sonia Lupien, a leading stress researcher from the University of Montreal, defines stress as "a state of imbalance between an individual's perceived demands and their perceived resources to cope with those demands." In other words, stress occurs when an individual feels overwhelmed by the challenges or demands they face, and believes they lack the necessary resources or coping mechanisms to deal with those challenges effectively.

Understanding *why* you experience stress is the first building block to becoming a resilient caregiver. Here, the keyword is "resilient." For Lupien, the opposite of stress is not serene bliss, but resilience. Although a relaxed state can temporarily help you cope with a stressful situation, it cannot permanently defuse your response to a repeated stressor. For this you must use a more creative approach in finding a lasting solution to a crisis that regularly pushes you beyond your limits.

With proper training, your brain can find one, two,...five, or dozens of creative solutions to address the same recurring stressor. Putting your brain to work makes you resilient. Resilience involves planning, making choices, and adapting. It's not innate, but it is a skill that caregivers can nurture through life experiences and various coping methods.

Dr. Lupien asserts that all stressful situations originate from one of four sources, embodied in the four letters of the acronym, **NUTS**. Let's uncover the four aspects of the NUTS framework and see how they can help us manage stress.

. . .

N - Novelty: You may feel stressed when you experience something new. What can you do to manage stress stemming from novelty?

- Gradually engage in new experiences to develop resilience toward novelty.
- Practice mindfulness and focus on the present moment to reduce the stress of the unknown.

U - Unpredictability: Stress may appear when there is no way of knowing what will happen. What can you do to manage stress stemming from unpredictability?

- Develop problem-solving skills to adapt to unexpected situations, analyzing the causes and triggers of your stress.
- Cultivate flexibility and an attitude of acceptance toward uncertainty. It's like surfing. You don't know the size of the next wave, so you develop techniques and strategies to surf waves of different sizes. This approach is how you come up with dozens of contingency plans.

T - Threatens your ego: Almost everyone experiences high stress levels when they feel their competency is being questioned. Stress related to a threat to the ego is closely connected to self-worth. When a situation or circumstance challenges your sense of competency, worth, or value, it can lead to feelings of inadequacy, self-doubt, and a drop in self-esteem. What can you do to manage stress stemming from a threat to the ego?

- Practice self-compassion and positive self-talk to manage self-esteem challenges.
- Seek support from friends, family, or a therapist to address feelings of inadequacy.
- Empower yourself with knowledge about your challenges.

S - Sense of control: Finally, you may experience stress when you are under the impression that you have little or no control over a situation. What can you do to manage stress stemming from a lack of control?

- Create a sense of structure by setting small achievable goals and prioritizing tasks.
- Use relaxation techniques such as deep breathing or meditation to manage feelings of helplessness.

To illustrate the NUTS acronym, let's take a closer look at Lovely and Jennifer's situation. Jennifer recognizes that caregiving can be overwhelming, and mentally prepares herself for it each day. So, what's causing her stress?

For Jennifer, the constant question from her mother about where her dad put the sewing machine really gets to her. When she examines this situation closely, she realizes that it's not just the repetition of the question; it's the painful reminder of her late father that stirs up her emotions. She understands that she can't control her father's passing, and the unpredictability of when her mother brings him up adds to her stress, touching on both the 'Sense of control' and 'Unpredictability' aspects of the NUTS acronym.

With this understanding, Jennifer can take a more compassionate approach by guiding her mother to discuss her sewing passion. By doing this, Jennifer can help her mother engage in the current conversation without bringing up the topic of her father. Knowing that Lovely will most likely ask the same question again, Jennifer might consider incorporating sewing-related activities into her mother's daily routine, perhaps twice a day.

To make a comparison, just as illnesses like COVID-19 can spread, stress can also have a contagious effect. However, in the same way we have measures to prevent infection, there are strategies to prevent stress from overwhelming us. Investing energy in reducing *your own* stress levels can significantly impact the anxiety of the person you're caring for. Additionally, it's essential to be mindful of how your loved one's stress can affect you. By identifying the sources of stress (in both you and your loved one) and taking simple steps to address those causes, you can diminish the spread. This proactive approach can stop the cycle of stress, bringing relief to you and your loved one with dementia.

YOUR WAY OUT OF GUILT

Caregiving is a demanding and often thankless job requiring significant time, energy, and emotional investment. Therefore, it is common for you as a caregiver to feel overwhelmed, stressed, and guilty about your experiences. Caregiver guilt can be incredibly challenging because it is often rooted in the belief that you're not doing enough for your loved one; when, in fact, you're doing everything you can, to the best of your ability, and with your loved one's best interests at heart.

Caring for someone with dementia intensifies these feelings due to the relentless demands for time and attention, often making caregivers feel inadequate. These emotions are normal in caregiving, underscoring the need for others to appreciate caregivers' remarkable dedication and compassion.

Below are the common types of guilt one might feel:

- Guilt for accidentally doing or saying something wrong
- Guilt for not being able to face the challenges of caregiving
- Guilt for bad emotions experienced while caring
- Guilt for being "selfish" when practicing self-care
- Guilt for ignoring other relatives

These feelings of guilt emerge when you start thinking that you are falling short in any or all of your roles and believe the relationship with your loved one is suffering. The reality is that to be a competent caregiver, you must also take care of yourself and let go of any feelings of guilt.

Here are a few ways to help you take more control of your emotions and learn to cope with caregiver guilt:

- **Practice self-compassion and affirmations**: Most times, you put the needs of your loved one before your own, but remember that taking care of yourself is just as important as taking care of your loved one. Practicing self-compassion can help you understand how to accept and forgive yourself, and will reduce feelings of guilt and burnout. **When repeated regularly and genuinely believed,** affirmations can be a powerfully **effective** tool to help you cope with guilt and maintain a positive mindset. Some good examples of affirmations would be:

"I prioritize self-care to better care for others."
"I am constantly learning and growing as a caregiver."
"I am strong and capable of handling the challenges of caregiving."
"I deserve support and am not afraid to ask for help when needed."
"I choose to focus on the moments of joy and connection in caregiving."
"I am taking things one step at a time and not overwhelming myself."
"I am grateful for the opportunity to provide love and support to my loved one."
"I acknowledge my own needs and take breaks when necessary."
"I am doing my best, and that is always enough."
"I embrace self-compassion and forgive myself for any perceived shortcomings."
"I choose to respond with patience and love."

- **Ask for help**: Caregiving can be a lonely experience; but remember, it's okay to ask for help. Whether from family members, friends, or community resources, reaching out for support can make a big difference in how you feel.
- **Set realistic expectations**: Caregiving can be a never-ending cycle of responsibilities and tasks. Set realistic expectations for yourself. By prioritizing tasks and focusing on what is most important, you can reduce feelings of guilt and prevent burnout. It may be helpful to write down your priorities and check them off one-by-one to offer yourself a small, yet gratifying, sense of accomplishment.
- **Connect with others**: Joining a support group or connecting with other caregivers can help give you a sense of community and validation. Talking to others who are going

through similar experiences as yourself can help to reduce feelings of guilt and increase feelings of self-worth. Refer to Chapter 7 for more details on support groups.

ELIMINATING CAREGIVER BURNOUT: DIAGNOSIS AND SOLUTIONS

Not much is intuitive when it comes to dementia care, but caregiving strategies can be taught and learned. Even healthcare professionals have to learn about dementia, the accompanying stress, and the system with which to minimize it.

Here are a few tell-tale signs of burnout:

1. **Constant stress**: Caregiving for someone with dementia can be a never-ending source of stress. The constant demands, the unpredictability of the situation, and the emotional toll of seeing a loved one's mind slowly decline can be overwhelming.
2. **Sleep disturbances**: Many caregivers experience disrupted sleep due to the demands of caregiving, which can lead to physical and emotional exhaustion.
3. **Neglecting self-care**: Caregivers often put their loved one's needs ahead of their own, neglecting self-care activities like exercise, hobbies, or even basic relaxation. This self-neglect can contribute to burnout.
4. **Helplessness and frustration**: Witnessing a loved one's cognitive and behavioral changes can evoke feelings of helplessness and frustration, as caregivers struggle to cope with challenging behaviors.
5. **Detachment**: Over time, the emotional toll can lead to a sense of detachment. Caregivers may become emotionally distant or even cynical about their caregiving role, losing the emotional connection they once had.
6. **Reduced self-esteem**: As burnout progresses, caregivers may feel like they're not doing a good job or failing their

loved one. It can result in lowered self-esteem and self-worth.

7. **Loss of motivation**: Constant stress and emotional strain can lead to a loss of motivation to persevere. Caregivers may feel like they're just going through the motions without the same care and compassion they had at the start.
8. **Physical symptoms**: Burnout appears through physical symptoms such as headaches, digestive issues, fatigue, muscle tension, lack of appetite, heart palpitations, changes in blood pressure, cognitive impairments, hair loss, weakened immune system, or even more severe health problems due to chronic stress.
9. **Increased irritability**: Caregivers experiencing burnout may become more irritable or easily frustrated, which can strain relationships with their loved ones and others.
10. **Isolation**: Burnout can lead to social withdrawal as caregivers may feel they don't have the time or energy to engage in social activities.

Note that burnout can vary from person to person, and not everyone will experience all of these signs. Healthcare providers may use formal assessments or interviews to diagnose and address burnout when working with caregivers and other individuals experiencing significant stress.

Fortunately, there are some ways to avoid burnout by reducing the stress you will likely experience as a caregiver:

- **Join a support group**: Joining a support group can be a helpful way for you to combat burnout because they provide space for caregivers to connect with others going through similar experiences, which can help alleviate feelings of isolation and loneliness. In Chapter 7, we will take an indepth look at support groups.
- **Seek empowerment**: Another way to address caregiver burnout is by seeking empowerment, which means taking steps to gain control over your situation. This strategy works

by educating yourself about your loved one with dementia's condition and treatment options. It is precisely what you are doing right now by reading this book. Education can empower you to feel more confident in providing care and making informed decisions.

- **Seek counseling**: Counseling provides a safe and confidential space for you as a caregiver to express your feelings and concerns. By working with a mental health professional, you can identify the root causes of your stress and develop strategies for managing it. Counseling can also help you learn coping skills, such as mindfulness and relaxation techniques, to help you manage stress levels and prevent burnout. It can also provide a supportive environment to process your emotions, such as anger, guilt, or frustration. We will talk more about counseling in Chapter 5.

Believe it or not, *your* stress and exhaustion can indirectly impact the well-being of your loved one. This is why I'm so eager to encourage you to prioritize self-care. Lending the best possible hand to yourself can help reduce the stress you experience from caring for your loved one with dementia. Adopting multiple coping strategies might actually help reduce your loved one's dementia symptoms and improve their overall well-being, not to mention your own. However, consulting a healthcare professional for personalized guidance and support is still important.

FIRST THINGS FIRST: CARE FOR YOURSELF

"Caregiving" is an actual "gift" to your loved one with dementia. But it is time-, resource-, and energy-consuming. You may think and say, as many dementia caregivers do, that you are fine and will take care of yourself later. But as can be demonstrated through research, **that's just not true**.

As we saw earlier, caregivers are more likely than others to develop chronic stress, depression, anxiety, cardiovascular problems, a weaker immune system, and a higher level of chronic conditions such as diabetes. Therefore, by caring for yourself, you'll preserve your health and, in essence, your loved one with dementia's health as well.

Caring for yourself doesn't mean spending lots of money or taking long vacations. Those are often unrealistic expectations. It's more about spending quality time alone, even just a few minutes, as often as possible. Small but consistent commitments to yourself daily will have a more significant impact in the long run than spending a whole day or week alone or away (although a day or week alone is also good).

And here's the secret: those small acts of self-care, when done regularly, add up to a happier, healthier you. There's so much to gain from spending short but regular self-care moments alone, such as strolling in your backyard or around the block, listening to one of your favorite songs, dancing to the beat, doing short strength or cardio training exercises, or practicing "mindfulness" (being "present" at what you do, when you do it). And if you're wondering what the long-term equation of this self-care is, I'll show you:

Little self-care activity + Consistency + Time
= Significant results on your well-being

Skipping them, on the other hand, can lead to a vicious cycle. For instance, if you skip your regular walks, you may start gaining weight, affecting your flexibility, agility, and self-esteem, which could make you not want to go out for a walk in public. On the contrary, if you take a walk, plant flowers, water the lawn, feed the birds, go to the park, sit on a bench, or cuddle with your dog for five minutes, it becomes your self-care moment—the moment you feel free and recharged with renewed energy.

CARE FOR YOURSELF ACCORDING TO YOUR PERSONALITY

As I have pointed out before, you can't take care of yourself enough. Due to the fact that we live in a deadline/productivity-driven society, caring for oneself is often an underdeveloped skill. However, you can only be productive if you're adequately energized and cared for.

We all have different preferences, life experiences, time schedules, and personalities, so you must discover what energizes you the most:

- To be around people or to be alone?
- To speak your feelings to others or let them fade away in silence or by listening to music?
- Are you an extrovert or an introvert?

Whichever one it is, be sure to do more of what fulfills you.

LANGUAGES OF LOVE: HOW YOU FEEL LOVED, HOW YOU SHOW LOVE

In his now-famous book, "5 Love Languages: The Secret to Love That Lasts", Gary Chapman introduces the concept of love languages, and breaks them down into five ways of expressing and receiving love in a relationship. This display of love comes in the form of: "words of affirmation, quality time, physical touch, acts of service, and giving/receiving gifts". Not everyone communicates love in the same manner; and different people prefer to receive love in different ways. So you must assess your own love language, and do more of those things that fill your heart with joy and satisfaction.

You may relate to most of these languages, but there's usually one that will resonate with you more than the others. I have put together a concise explanation of each one for you to discover which love language fits you best.

Acts Of Service

If acts of service is your love language, then you feel that actions more valuable than words. You appreciate it more when someone does extra effort to make things easy—bringing you soup while sick or making coffee for you in the morning are good examples.

• • •

Receiving Gifts

People in this category respond to visual indicators of love. They value the present itself, and the giver's time and effort in picking it out. To them, that is what shows affection and love.

Quality Time

Individuals whose love language falls in this category want undivided attention. They feel loved when their loved one is present and focused on them. Examples are turning off the computer, putting down the phone, making eye contact, and genuinely listening.

Words Of Affirmation

Individuals in this group value verbal acknowledgments, compliments, words of appreciation, and emotional encouragement. They also appreciate messaging or social media engagement.

Physical Touch

When someone's primary love language is physical contact, they feel love through physical affection. Besides sex, they feel loved when their partner holds their hand, strokes their arm, hugs them, or massages them after a long day.

If you still can't determine which love language speaks to you the most, you can take the quiz at https://5lovelanguages.com/quizzes/love-language. Knowing your primary love language might help you complete the next exercise more easily. In the following table, I have included a few activities to help you care for yourself in less than ten minutes a day. Take two or three minutes to go through the table and journal about your preferred daily self-care practice. It can help you be more present in what you do for yourself and take you one step further from your daily care-related challenges. All you have to do is choose an activity.

MORE JOY AND PEACE IN LESS THAN 10 MINS., ACCORDING TO YOUR LOVE LANGUAGE

SELFCARE ACTIVITIES	ACT OF SERVICE	GIFT	QUALITY TIME	WORDS OF AFFIRMATION	PHYSICAL TOUCH
Take 3 to 10 breaths					X
Stretch					X
Dance					X
Exercise					X
Hug someone					X
Drop your shoulders					X
Self massage			X		X
Walk			X		X
Moisturize	X				X
Message a friend	X			X	
Drink 2 glasses of water several times during the day	X				X
Look at the sky or scenery and be present	X		X		
Pet your dog or cat			X		X
Accept a compliment			X	X	

SELFCARE ACTIVITIES	ACT OF SERVICE	GIFT	QUALITY TIME	WORDS OF AFFIRMATION	PHYSICAL TOUCH
Pray			X	X	
Quality time with a friend			X		
Practice mindfulness			X		
Laugh			X	X	
Read a good book		X	X	X	
Draw			X		
Play or listen to music			X		
Drink a cup of tea, coffee or fresh juice		X	X		X
Light a candle		X	X		
Journal		X		X	
Make an affirmation. Believe what you say.				X	
Buy yourself a special item		X			
Drive on a peaceful road	X		X		

WHEN YOU NEED TO CONSULT A PROFESSIONAL

QUESTIONS	NEVER	SOMETIMES	OFTEN
Do you have trouble going to sleep?			
Do you usually get up at night?			
Do your dreams cause you any stress?			
Do you have anxiety or panic attacks?			
Have you experienced significant weight loss or gain in the past few weeks or months?			
Do you frequently endure illnesses like recurring colds, the flu, or soar throats?			
Have you started experiencing persistent health issues like high blood pressure, headaches, or backaches?			
Do small annoyances or irritations often lead you to tears/anger?			
Do you feel that your situation is hopeless?			
Have you given up any enjoyable hobbies or interests?			
Do you interact with people less frequently?			
Does caring affect your career?			

Answering the previous questions by selecting "never," "sometimes," or "often" will help you decide whether you need professional help or not.

As a caregiver, you must prioritize your mental health and seek support when needed. If your responses leaned toward 'sometimes' or 'often' for most of these questions, it might indicate the necessity for support in managing the care of your loved one with dementia *while* prioritizing your own well-being. Consider including others in the caregiving role, no matter how close you are to your loved one. Caregiving involves a range of responsibilities. Sharing these responsibilities will help you and your loved one have a better quality of life.

The learning process is only complete once the acquired knowledge is put to good use. Therefore, I strongly encourage you to apply the ideas we have studied so far.

Any progress is BIG PROGRESS. One step at a time.

We've just delved into valuable insights about self-care for dementia caregivers and practical tips to manage stress, avoid burnout, and enhance your well-being. Now, let's take another compassionate step forward.

As we journey together through this book, strengthening trust in your caregiving abilities is at the core of our exploration. So, in the upcoming chapter, we'll immerse ourselves in the world of your loved one with dementia. By gaining a deeper understanding of their experiences, you'll be able to notice things more closely and come up with better ways to help them. It will make your caregiving journey more meaningful, and aid you in connecting to your loved one's needs.

CHAPTER 3
IN YOUR LOVED ONE'S SHOES

In every Alzheimer's story, there is also a love story. Hold onto yours, for it can carry you and your loved one through the longest days and darkest nights.

-Rosalys Peel, author of *Mike & Me*

As time passed, Lovely's condition continued deteriorating. She became mostly gloomy and increasingly frustrated with occasional scary moments and threatening behavior. "Mom is terrified, and wants to 'go home,'" Jennifer said, "She walks to the door as if she knows where to go and looks around the house like she's looking for something. Then demands to see her own mother or her husband; but they've both been dead for a while now."

Jennifer kept telling her that Dad and Grandma were no longer alive, but Lovely didn't seem interested in what her daughter said. The only thing she seemed concerned about was not falling while pacing around the house.

Although she was very mobile, Lovely's perception was no longer what it used to be. As her condition progressed, Jennifer had to ensure her mom was kept safe and well cared for. Even when Jennifer was tired, she couldn't leave her mom alone, otherwise Lovely might try to leave the house and stroll into danger. So, she had to adopt various strategies to keep her mom at home. Jennifer installed locks and cowbells on the doors and started hiding Lovely's shoes. "Mom would only go out of the house with her shoes on," she said.

HOW DEMENTIA AFFECTS YOUR LOVED ONE'S PERCEPTION

When your loved one is diagnosed with dementia, their experience changes how they perceive things. As dementia progresses, the way they experience the world around them changes as well. These changes may include:

- Misperceptions (wrong interpretation)
- Misidentifications (believing one person to be someone else)
- Hallucinations (hearing and seeing things that appear to be real but are not)
- Delusions (having a clearly false belief)
- Time-shifting (re-living the past)

This is because, as stated earlier, dementia targets and damages specific parts of the brain, which causes the person to understand things differently. When information is picked up by the sense organs, such as the eyes, ears, or tongue, it is transmitted to the brain. The brain processes this information for it to be understood. The brain analyzes the incoming information with other stored data, such as thoughts, memories, and emotions linked to the sensory input. The individual then becomes aware of what has been sensed.

Dementia can disrupt this process, altering how your loved one perceives the world around them. These disruptions can result from damage to the eyes or portions of the brain, and can lead to the person with dementia saying or doing things that make no sense to anyone but themselves. This can be frustrating, confusing, and unpleasant for others, particularly caregivers who spend the most time with them.

WHY YOUR LOVED ONE WITH DEMENTIA ACTS THE WAY THEY DO

A person recently diagnosed with dementia is likely to experience a wide range of emotions. Grief, loss, rage, shock, terror, disbelief, and even relief are a few examples. The lack of proper control over these emotions can result in unusual reactions that you, as the caregiver, will have to witness.

Some of the causes for these actions could be the following:

- **Emotional effects**: People who have dementia frequently experience alterations in their emotional responses. They may have less control over how they communicate their feelings. For example, your loved one may overreact to situations or suffer quick mood swings. Caregivers commonly find it difficult to deal with these sudden changes. It is worth remembering that they are partly caused by damage done to the brain.
- **Impact on confidence and self-esteem**: People with dementia are more likely to feel uneasy and lose confidence in themselves and their abilities. They may feel out of control and lose faith in their own judgment. As a result of their diagnosis, they may also face external stigma and "social demotion." Social demotion is when someone's status or position in society decreases or becomes lower than it was before (i.e. they are offered different respect, opportunities, or privileges than they were previously used to).

I'll advise you, the caregiver, to avoid harsh criticism or belittling comments at the time when your loved one acts irrationally. Don't judge yourself if you acted this way in the past. You did the best you could with what you knew, and if you are reading this now, it means you want to keep learning because you deeply care about your loved one.

Although dementia is a degenerative condition, some capacities will remain almost intact until the end. Memory of prayers, music, and poetry are some of these enduring talents because they are associated with emotional centers in the brain. These prevailing abilities are crucial for entering into the world of your loved one.

To simplify the analysis of the day-to-day effects of dementia and how they change the perspective of your loved one's life, I have opted to use the 3-stage model instead of the Global Deterioration Scale (the 7-stage model).

THE 3 STAGES OF DEMENTIA, AND HOW YOUR LOVED ONE MAY FEEL AT EACH STAGE

STAGE 1 - Early stage (mild)

In early-stage dementia, some days may be symptom-free, but behaviors gradually become more constant. Anxiety is generally common at this point, since your loved one is still aware of their losses and may attempt to conceal them.

- **Mild memory losses**: In Alzheimer's disease and vascular dementia, mild memory loss may cause trouble in the everyday life of your loved one with dementia. In general, your loved one will still be aware of these memory losses, but focusing on them does not help. It is better to avoid "testing" the memory of your loved one with dementia. Instead, please encourage them to find other strategies such as a notebook, sticky pads, pill organizers for their medication, establishing routines, etc. In the early stage of Alzheimer's disease, your loved one may forget where to go when they are out; they may also forget appointments, or how to dress accordingly with the current weather; they may omit paying bills, or forget their favorite recipes or hobbies. Because short-term memory loss can be so frightening, your loved one may react strongly to deny it. For example, they may try to hide it from you or attempt to compensate with abilities not yet impaired by the neurodegeneration process.
- **Misplacing objects**: Due to their memory loss, your loved one with dementia may frequently misplace things, such as

common items in the kitchen, keys, glasses, or cutlery. They may put something away for safekeeping and then forget where it is. They may also leave objects in strange places, such as the TV remote control in the bathroom or tea bags in the refrigerator. If your loved one expects an item to be somewhere, but it isn't, they may suspect that someone is hiding their things or stealing from them. Your loved one may attempt to regain control of their circumstances by hiding or hoarding their belongings, hence the urge to stockpile items.

- **Loss of motor coordination**: Your loved one with dementia may be unable to perform certain tasks or purposeful movements when asked, even though they A) understand the request, B) are willing to complete the task, C) have the muscles needed to perform it correctly, and D) have already learned how to do the task before. They may also experience difficulties with balance, dressing themselves, holding objects, or handwriting. Doctors call this "apraxia," which refers to impaired communication between the brain and muscles.
- **Sleep Disturbances:** Your loved one may experience mild sleep disruptions, including insomnia, nighttime awakenings, and difficulties distinguishing day from night. Restlessness and occasional sleep-related behaviors may also occur.
- **Difficulty understanding complex documents**: Your loved one with dementia may need help understanding financial records and managing their budget. As a result, they may quickly become a target of scammers and need help to distinguish deception.
- **Difficulty following multi-step instructions**: Your loved one might encounter difficulty completing tasks, possibly starting one thing and then shifting to another halfway through. Tasks that were previously effortless, like following instructions, could now pose significant challenges for them.

- **Difficulty managing finances:** Some individuals might encounter difficulties in managing finances, but it's not a constant issue, yet.
- **Difficulty with planning and organization:** Planning and organization skills might start to decline, leading to occasional difficulties in these areas.
- **Lost in conversations**: They may get lost during a conversation and have difficulty finding their words.
- **Repeating sentences or questions**: Although it may be very annoying, repetition is a way for your loved one with dementia to feel secure. They may not remember immediate conversations, making a loop with the same sentence or question.
- **Impossible to keep their job**: Because of the cognitive impairments detailed above, your loved one with dementia might lose their job if they show even one of them, or their employer might ask them to retire. In this circumstance, a social worker or counselor can help navigate this challenging situation. I will elaborate more on this in Chapter 5, but a social worker will attempt to verify if dementia is the leading cause of your loved one's performance decline at work, and will help them get all the necessary benefits and financial assistance from the federal government.
- **Communication challenges**: From the early stages, your loved one with dementia might start substituting simple words, for instance, saying "the thing where I sit" instead of "chair." They may also shorten their sentences to avoid words they don't remember. For instance, they might say "fridge milk " instead of "Can I have some cold milk?" With the sentence "fridge milk," a person with dementia may not be attempting to express the word "fridge" but rather the concept of "cold." The challenge may lie in their inability to articulate the word "cold," so they substitute it with "fridge," a term they recognize as being associated with coldness. Put

yourself in your loved one's shoes for a moment: imagine you are learning a foreign language, and you can't find the exact word for an idea. Just like all of us do in such situations, you resort to a description or different word that means almost the same thing to convey the intended meaning effectively. Looking for the right word without finding it can understandably make them upset or very emotional, especially if you or someone else brings up the issue.

- **Swearing or cursing:** Because dementia affects your loved one's ability to think, communicate, and perform daily activities, at this stage, your loved one may experience changes in their verbal behavior too, including the increased use of swear words. One reason for this behavior change could be that the parts of the brain responsible for language and social norms are affected by dementia. As a result, your loved one may struggle to control their language. Sometimes, articulating "normal" words and phrases may be challenging, while inappropriate language might come quickly. The reason for this apparent paradox may be that the part of the brain responsible for "normal" language could be affected by dementia, while the one for swear words might not be. It's just helpful to know they're probably not doing it on purpose.
- **Spatial orientation and challenges with driving**: It may become impossible for your loved one to drive at this stage because of the risk of getting lost or because they have difficulties evaluating distances between objects, especially in the presence of backgrounds identically colored to the objects they are trying to focus on.
- **Lack of spatial awareness**: Your loved one with dementia might be unable to differentiate a carpet from the floor if there is not enough of a contrast. This may represent a fall risk.
- **Lack of time awareness**: Your loved one with dementia might completely lose track of time. Their internal

(biological) clock might be disturbed because of neurodegeneration.

- **Sundowning**: You may notice changes in your loved one's behavior later in the afternoon or near the end of the day. During this time, your loved one may become extremely upset and anxious, or start to have hallucinations or delusions. This may persist throughout the night, making it difficult for them to sleep. The phenomenon is called "sundowning," and the exact causes are still unknown to this day. It might result from a disturbance of the body's biological clock; but some other possible causes include tiredness, boredom, and pain.
- **Depression** is a common symptom in the early stages of dementia and may be an early warning sign that your loved one is developing the condition. As a caregiver, you must know the connection between the two. When your loved one realizes they are losing their abilities, they might begin feeling useless and ashamed of their incapacities, and depression may start to manifest.
- **Visual or auditory hallucinations:** Your loved one might feel, smell, see, or hear something that does not exist. Hallucinations are symptoms that can come and go. When they believe they are witnessing a frightening or dangerous scenario, object, or person, your loved one with dementia may become terrified. On the contrary, they might hallucinate more pleasant realities and actually enjoy them. Either situation may be disturbing or scary for caregivers as they might feel their loved one with dementia is "going crazy." Again, brain damage can cause that kind of altered perception. Sadly, this particular symptom might make it difficult to find respite care services adapted to your loved one's needs when you require a break. For instance, daycare centers generally work with groups. Thus, many may reject your loved one's application because their staff does not have sufficient time or training to handle situations induced by psychosis-like symptoms. Be patient and persevere. The

"For Caregivers" section of the NADSA website has resources that may help you find a special daycare for your loved one.

- **Agnosia** is the term used to describe a persistent lack of recognition of individuals or objects. The brain can no longer interpret the signals (shapes, faces, sounds, smells) that the senses deliver.
- **Mood swings** in dementia can manifest as impulsive behavior, mood, and personality changes. Your loved one may be irritated, depressed, anxious, or agitated. These mood changes can occur without warning, but usually only last for a short time.
- **Denial and anosognosia:** You will notice your loved one denying that they have a problem with memory loss or changes in their thinking abilities. They may refuse to seek medical attention or participate in activities that would help diagnose or manage their condition. They could have any number of reasons or excuses, including fear of the unknown, difficulty accepting the diagnosis, and a lack of understanding of the condition. Anosognosia is a term used to describe the condition in which an individual cannot recognize their own physical or mental health problems or disabilities. This lack of awareness makes the caregiver's task particularly challenging, as individuals with dementia may, at times, refuse treatment or care due to their inability to perceive themselves as being sick. In such situations, engaging in arguments with your loved one over their diagnosis becomes futile as they consistently fail to acknowledge it, leading to repetitive and unproductive discussions. If your loved one refuses to take their required medication, you may need to improvise and try strategies such as mixing their medicine with a meal they like. I will get back to such methods in more detail in Chapter 4.

STAGE 2– Middle stage (moderate)

In this phase, other people start noticing some differences in your loved one's thinking. Still, these differences are usually not too substantial, and might not cause significant disruptions in their everyday activities.

- **Memory loss:** Memory loss and difficulty thinking get worse. Your loved one with dementia might get close relatives mixed up with strangers. They may forget names, details, and recent events. It may be impossible for them to learn new things. In a desperate attempt to do so, they might ask the same question over and over again.
- **Self-awareness:** Your loved one's self-awareness might still be well preserved at this stage. In fact, self-awareness can be preserved even in the severe stage of dementia. As long as the regions of the brain associated with self-awareness remain safe from neurodegeneration, your loved one may not understand why caregivers, healthcare providers, or close relatives talk and act as if they are not in the same room. They may feel as though they are being ignored, and find it very difficult from an emotional standpoint to witness.
- **Sleep Disruptions:** During the middle stage of dementia, sleep disturbances tend to intensify. Fragmented sleep, nighttime wandering, daytime sleepiness may become prominent. Sleep disorders, like sleep apnea, may develop.
- **Language challenges:** Language impairments worsen as well in this stage. Your loved one with dementia might have trouble finding their words, and they might stop speaking in the middle of a sentence because they forgot what they wanted to say.
- **Agitation and aggression:** Mood swings become more intense. Your loved one might become agitated and, in some cases, aggressive, often triggered by confusion or frustration. It is key to understand that agitation, like other behavioral and psychological symptoms of dementia, *always* has an underlying cause such as physical discomfort, overstimulation (e.g. loud noises, large groups of unfamiliar

people, being asked too many questions, or confronted with too complex a task), boredom, etc.

- **Behavioral changes:** Symptoms of apathy, depression, and anxiety might persist in this stage. Sudden mood swings are common. In the case of Frontotemporal dementia, saying inappropriate things, stealing, or even undressing in public is possible.
- **Inappropriate sexual behaviors:** Though it is uncommon in the dementia population, it does happen. Inappropriate sexual behaviors are caused by brain impairment, not your loved one's desire to exhibit themselves. Sometimes, your loved one might simply confuse someone with their spouse due to the damage done by their dementia. When redirected gently with no judgment, a mild reaction will probably happen instead of getting upset for feeling rejected.
- **Wandering:** This results from feeling lost or perhaps looking for someone or something. It is an uncontrollable behavior that can happen in either a familiar location or a new environment; although changes of environment commonly increase this behavior. When wandering occurs, 24/7 supervision is necessary as your loved one could potentially get lost anytime during the day or night.
- **Shadowing:** Shadowing refers to a behavior where your loved one with dementia follows you, their caregiver, or another loved one around, frequently standing or walking close behind. This occurs because you might be the only stable landmark for your loved one with dementia, which results in constantly following you in order to feel safe.

STAGE 3 – Late stage (severe)

- **Full-time support**: In late-stage dementia, your loved one gradually requires full-time support in almost all tasks of daily living and personal care. They might fall if they try to walk as their brain no longer controls their muscles correctly. It gradually becomes almost impossible to talk, eat, swallow, walk, bathe, go to the bathroom, or even control their bladder and bowel movements. On top of that, their perception of reality becomes altered as well.

- **Deteriorating memory**: Your loved one with dementia might live in the past as memory problems worsen. They may think they are at an earlier time of their life and ask for long-gone "significant others" from their past. They may no longer recognize familiar people and places. It could even go as far as not recognizing themselves when they look in the mirror, potentially because they might be expecting to see a younger version of themself.
- **Speaking is difficult**: The language abilities of your loved one with dementia may gradually disappear until only a few words of their mother tongue remain. Dementia might also significantly impair their understanding, but their abilities to recognize gestures and facial expressions generally remain.
- **Physical challenges**: Gait may be slow and unsteady; eventually, your loved one with dementia might need a wheelchair to avoid falls. Appetite goes down, and difficulties swallowing and eating trigger weight loss and weakness.
- **Weakness**: Poor food intake and absence of movement increase the risk of strokes and blood clots, a common cause of death in late-stage dementia.
- **Vulnerability to infections**: Vulnerability to infections can be a sign of advanced dementia, particularly in the late stages. As dementia progresses, it can affect a person's immune system and ability to fight off infections, leading to increased susceptibility to illnesses such as pneumonia. Pneumonia is a severe lung infection that can cause prolonged coughing, difficulty breathing, and chest pain. In people with dementia, pneumonia can potentially be life-threatening. Recognizing the symptoms of pneumonia might be difficult, mainly because your loved one generally has trouble communicating. To prevent pneumonia, preserving your loved one's overall health and well-being is essential,

particularly by maintaining good hygiene, like regular hand washing, practicing proper nutrition, and avoiding exposure to infections.

CATASTROPHIC REACTIONS AND AGGRESSIONS

Contrary to other behaviors, catastrophic reactions can happen at any stage. A catastrophic reaction is an overreaction to a seemingly normal, non-threatening situation, sometimes accompanied by physically acting-out in a way that seems inappropriate or out of proportion to the problem. It is sometimes called a "rage reaction", and is characterized by an excessive and sudden emotional response or physical behavior. The trigger for a catastrophic reaction can vary. Often, the individual with dementia might not feel well or could feel hurried and disoriented. At times, it may stem from numerous small occurrences throughout the day, such as fleeting moments of confusion, correction, or frustration that culminate in an outburst later in the day. Catastrophic reactions present themselves as sudden angry outbursts, verbal aggression (for example, shouting and cursing), threats or even acts of physical aggression, such as hitting, kicking, and biting. These types of aggressive reactions can be considered an outcome of psychological disturbances.

Encountering aggression doesn't necessarily imply helplessness in controlling the situation. It typically stems from triggers that can be minimized and stressors that can be alleviated, such as loud environments, physical discomfort, disruptions in routine, boredom, and more. These non-pharmaceutical approaches are very effective in preventing aggressivity and aggression. Professionals can help you find more strategies like these without the need to prescribe antipsychotics. In fact, recent research shows limited effects, and many adverse side effects, of medication on these types of behaviors.

BEING SICK IN ADDITION TO DEMENTIA

People with dementia are already vulnerable. For instance, poor balance can come with aging, causing a greater risk of falling. Your loved one with dementia may have fallen during the day, not remembered it, and kept functioning with a fracture. A benign condition can quickly worsen since your loved one cannot express pain or sensations clearly. Your loved one may catch the flu and feel disoriented or agitated. Wounds or bedsores may appear on their skin, get infected, and cause fever. Or, your loved one's teeth may hurt because of an abscess that never came up in conversation.

Your loved one's mobility might undergo changes as well. For instance, they may reduce their walking due to a foot problem, but they may forget to communicate this issue or struggle to express themselves. They might also experience nutritional deficiencies, dehydration, or have unhealthy eating habits. These factors may contribute to the development of delirium, consequently exacerbating their behavior. When delirium arises, the task of caring for your loved one with dementia can become notably more demanding. Therefore, further elaboration on this condition is required.

What is Delirium?

Delirium is a set of symptoms that alters consciousness, thinking, memory, physical activity, perception, and emotional state. It is associated with a sudden change in your loved one's thinking, awareness, and behavior, triggered by factors like dehydration, urinary tract infections, certain medications, or metabolic disorders. In older adults, delirium can significantly increase the risk of serious health problems and, in some cases, even be life-threatening.

Recognizing Delirium

Delirium often presents itself through varying motor behaviors, ranging from heightened activity (restlessness) to reduced activity (lethargy). Delirium is categorized into three subtypes based on motor activity: hyperactive, hypoactive, and mixed. Additionally, delirium can manifest as disturbances in the sleep-wake cycle, confusion, disorientation, agitation, hallucinations, or mood swings. What sets delirium apart from other conditions is that these symptoms fluctuate and may swiftly worsen, particularly at night.

Distinguishing Delirium from Dementia

Delirium differs from dementia in its rapid onset, often occurring within days, and in the fluctuating nature of its symptoms. Dementia, on the other hand, typically develops slowly over several months, except for cases of dementia with Lewy bodies (DLB). Research suggests there might be a strong connection between delirium and DLB, making it difficult to differentiate between the two. Individuals with DLB seem more susceptible to delirium than those with other types of dementia though. And other findings suggest that delirium may be an early sign of dementia with Lewy bodies. However, further research is needed to confirm this connection.

Why Early Detection of Delirium Matters

Early recognition of delirium is vital. As explained above, delirium can be caused by several factors, some of which are acute conditions that require immediate medical attention. When delirium is identified early, the underlying cause can be addressed, and appropriate treatment can be initiated. A timely intervention can help prevent complications, reduce suffering, and improve the chances of full recovery. Thus, if you notice *abrupt* changes in motor activity, behavior, or confusion, seek medical attention immediately. The timeliness of your intervention can save your loved one's life.

Prevention

The following tips are directly designed to address the potential causes of delirium (dehydration, urinary tract infections, certain medications, and metabolic disorders). To help prevent delirium, ensure your loved one stays hydrated, keep an updated list of their medications, and encourage a balanced diet and exercise.

I hope this subsection gave you valuable insights into delirium and its differences with dementia. Your efforts are not in vain, and your dedication may tremendously impact your loved one's life. Now, let's briefly conclude this section on the stages of dementia.

Please remember that the specific type of dementia your loved one has, and their unique situation will affect what they go through. It's not a one-size-fits-all approach, but these stages and symptoms give us an idea of where they might be in their dementia journey. With that in mind, I'd like to invite you to step into their shoes and try to understand what your loved one might be feeling.

WALK A MILE IN YOUR LOVED ONE'S SHOES: PRACTICAL EXERCISES

Life is a tapestry of emotions, shaping our experiences and interactions with the world around us. Understanding these emotions and empathizing with what others feel is a cornerstone of human connection. It's like having a window into someone's soul, allowing us to comprehend their actions and behaviors more deeply. When we extend this understanding to our loved one with dementia, whose behaviors can often be puzzling or perplexing, it becomes even more significant.

For individuals with dementia, communicating their needs and emotions can be an uphill battle. Their behaviors often serve as a form of expression, revealing their internal state. Challenging behaviors can be a way for them to convey distress, anxiety, or unmet needs, which they struggle to articulate conventionally. In such moments, it's crucial to view their actions through the lens of their emotions, realizing that their behavior is a response to what they're feeling inside.

To truly grasp what your loved one with dementia experiences, you can attempt to put yourself in their shoes. Here are some exercises you can do, ideally with a partner, to simulate what your loved one might feel. If you aren't able to practice with someone else, try to imagine how you would feel in the various situations listed. This understanding can help you provide better care and support to your loved one, especially during challenging times.

MEALTIME		
Roleplay activity: If it was you?	**How do you feel after the activity?**	**What your loved one may experience**
1-Be fed by someone who does not speak to you.		Your loved one with dementia may feel isolation
2-Be fed by someone who doesn't look you in the eyes and is talking to someone else.		Your loved one with dementia may not feel considered because of their lack of competencies
3-Be fed with something without knowing what it is.		Your loved one with dementia may feel lost because of brain damage
4-Be fed while pinching your nose shut.		The effects of neurodegeneration can significantly impact your loved one's senses and perceptions. It may include: • Smell • Taste • Delusions about food • Swallowing difficulties • Poor hand-to-mouth coordination • Oral/dental problems • Increased side effects from medications, etc.

ELIMINATION		
Roleplay activity: If it was you?	**How do you feel after the activity?**	**What your loved one may experience**
1-What would you think if I came up to you now and asked you to go to the toilet with me?		Your loved one with dementia may feel forced to do what they can't do.
2-What if you needed the toilet and couldn't find it?		Your loved one with dementia may feel panicked about urinating or defecating in their pants

HEARING PROBLEMS		
Roleplay activity: If it was you?	**How do you feel after the activity?**	**What your loved one may experience**
Put in earplugs and try to write down what someone is telling you in a normal tone of voice		Your loved one with dementia may have trouble focusing on your instructions during an activity.

VISION PROBLEMS		
Roleplay activity: If it was you?	**How do you feel after the activity?**	**What your loved one may experience**
1-Put on swimming goggles and read a paragraph from a newspaper or a book		Your loved one with dementia may not see correctly, feel frustrated or too proud to ask for help.
2-Put on swimming goggles and brush your teeth		Because of vision problems, basic activities of daily living become hard to execute. This could explain your loved one's reluctance to perform those tasks.
DISORIENTATION		
Roleplay activity: If it was you?	**How do you feel after the activity?**	**What your loved one may experience**
1-Have you ever woken up and struggled to find out where you were?		Your loved one with dementia may constantly feel lost in space.
2-What if you were meeting with a stranger in your house every day of the year?		Your loved one with dementia may feel afraid, or disturbed by someone they consider a stranger.

DISINHIBITION		
Roleplay activity: If it was you?	**How do you feel after the activity?**	**What your loved one may experience**
1-Do you ever have fantasies you never enact (especially sexual ones)?		Your loved one with dementia may not be able to keep their fantasies in their mind, may not know the difference between imagination and reality.
2-When angry, do you think of things you want to do but never will do?		Your loved one with dementia may not be able to stop the burst of anger, or filter slurs.
COMMUNICATION		
Roleplay activity: If it was you?	**How do you feel after the activity?**	**What your loved one may experience**
1-Ask someone to give you seven instructions without stopping.		Your loved one with dementia may feel overwhelmed, ignored or bullied.
2-Ask someone to give you these seven instructions one at a time but frowning, with an authoritarian tone and crossed arms.		Your loved one with dementia may refuse to listen to the message if your non-verbal communication is aggressive and condescending.

Understanding all the changes that can occur in your loved one's journey with dementia can indeed feel overwhelming. I genuinely respect your determination to learn and find solutions.

In the upcoming chapter, we'll continue our journey of discovery, where you'll find valuable insights and get a better grasp of what you can influence and control.

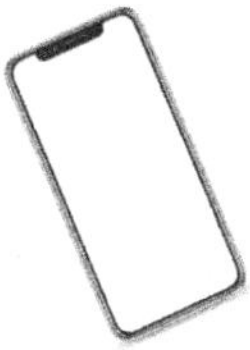

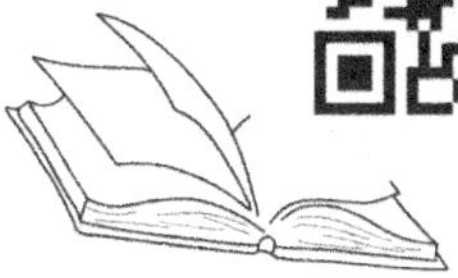

CHAPTER 4

WHAT YOU CAN CONTROL

"K*indness can transform someone's dark moment with a blaze of light. You'll never know how much your caring matters."*

-Amy Leigh Mercree

"With the last tap, Mom woke from her longest hours of sleep this week. Over the past few days, she has been more awake and conscious than allowing herself to rest. Although she has been acting weird, she's not violent for now, nor does she create a scene. Still, through observations, I have noticed that Mom is affected by noisy and crowded environments. As a result, I avoid taking her to crowded and noisy places and limit her social life to immediate family and a small circle of close and old friends," Jennifer wrote in her journal.

Sometimes, Jennifer would find her mother in front of the mirror, talking to her image. It would be nearly impossible to convince Lovely to leave the mirror, let alone the room, as she claimed she 'had company'. After a few incidents, Jennifer learned that there was no point in aggressively threatening her mother, but to play along, sometimes even joining her mom in the mirror conversation. After all, being a caregiver requires patience and understanding. You need to empathize with them and visualize yourself in the shoes of your loved one with dementia to make them feel understood.

Sometimes, Lovely believed she was in her cousin's house and couldn't find her belongings. Jennifer had to learn how to apply active strategies in order to enter her mom's world. At times like this, she might say, "You're right, Mom. I'll ask your cousin where your things are. I'm sure she knows where they are. I'm here with you. You're safe."

Caring for your loved one with dementia can indeed be challenging and stressful. But with the right approach, it can be a rewarding and even satisfying experience. This chapter will examine how to use the humanistic, resource-oriented approach in caring for your loved one with dementia. You will also discover "care strategies" to maintain balance in your relationship with them, especially as symptoms get worse along the stages of dementia. Note that the ideas shared in this chapter are solely my approach to dementia as a care provider, and should not be considered professional medical advice.

DELVING INTO HUMANISTIC APPROACHES: ADDING VALUE TO HUMAN POTENTIAL

In dementia caregiving, theoretical concepts may seem like distant academic ideas. However, as you'll soon discover, they hold practical keys to enhancing your daily caregiving experiences with your loved one.

1. Humanistic and Person-Centered Approaches (Brian Abrams, Carl Rogers): Empowering Your Loved One with Dementia Through Compassion and Connection

- **Explanation:** Humanistic and person-centered approaches recognize that all individuals have innate capacities for pursuing health and well-being. This perspective emphasizes the intrinsic value of selfhood, hope, creativity, and authenticity, which are integral to well-being. It shifts away from viewing individuals solely through the lens of their condition. Instead, it fosters a therapeutic environment built on empathy, unconditional acceptance, and trustworthiness.

- **Illustration:** Rather than focusing solely on your loved one's condition, you approach them with genuine understanding and acceptance. For example, if your loved one with dementia wanders, try to understand what they need before trying to stop them. For instance, if they say they must go home because they have work to do, it might mean they want to feel useful. Feeling active is a profoundly human need. Your loved one with dementia is no different.

2. Resource-Oriented Approach (Randi Rolvsjord): Recognizing and Nurturing Your Loved One's Strengths

- **Explanation:** As discussed by Randi Rolvsjord, the resource-oriented approach emphasizes the importance of identifying and nurturing your loved one's strengths and abilities. These strengths encompass their unique talents, creativity, and individuality, all of which contribute to their overall well-being. This perspective encourages caregivers to recognize and support their loved one's innate capabilities.
- **Illustration:** Despite your loved one's challenges, you discover their hidden talents, such as creating art or sharing stories from their past. By nurturing these strengths, you provide opportunities for self-expression and fulfillment, showcasing the power of strength-based caregiving.

3. Brain Pathways Activation (Boso et al.): Awakening Memories and Emotions Through Music

- **Explanation:** Music can remarkably activate specific brain pathways associated with emotions and memories, even when verbal communication is limited. Music stimulates emotional responses and facilitates meaningful connections with individuals living with dementia.

- **Illustration:** Imagine your loved one, who often appears distant and unresponsive. Playing a cherished song from their past brings tears to their eyes, rekindling memories and allowing them to communicate emotions without words. Music's ability to awaken these pathways offers precious moments of connection and reminiscence.

4. Preservation of Memory with Familiar Music (Cuddy and Duffin): Creating Joyous Moments of Connection

- **Explanation:** Familiar music possesses a unique capacity to preserve memory and prompt motor activity, providing opportunities for meaningful interactions with individuals living with dementia. This preservation of memory through music creates moments of joy and connection.
- **Illustration:** Picture your loved one, who may struggle to recognize family members, suddenly singing along to a beloved childhood song. As they hum each note, you witness the profound power of familiar music in preserving memory and fostering joyful connections between your loved one and those around them.

5. Connection and Relationship-Centered Care (Freud, Rio): Fostering Deep Bonds and Emotional Support

- **Explanation:** Connection and relationship-centered care, based on the ideas of "therapeutic alliance" by Freud, focuses on trust, empathy, and open communication between caregivers and their loved ones with dementia. It goes beyond regular caregiving, creating trust, understanding, and emotional support. It also highlights the value of connecting with others in the community. You could consider joining a support group of fellow dementia caregivers and their loved ones to build trust, empathy, and communication outside your home. A support group helps share memories and emotions openly and make profound connections. Being part of such a group is like finding a second family that genuinely understands what you are going through.

- **Illustration:** When your loved one with dementia is experiencing distressing delusions and disorientation, your calm and understanding presence gives them a sense of safety and reassurance, even if they constantly exhibit confusion regarding their surroundings or identity. Likewise, there are countless benefits to joining a community-based music therapy support group for caregivers and their loved ones with dementia. In a 2018 study by Robin Rio at Arizona State University, a group member shared their experience within this supportive community: "We come together weekly from all over the county, some traveling an hour to get there. Yet we all make an effort every week because we have become close friends and love singing together and sharing our memories and feelings with one another..."

These examples highlight the significance of empathy within your caregiving journey, and the potential for meaningful connections with others who understand your experiences as dementia caregivers. Such alliances can provide invaluable support and a sense of belonging during these challenging times.

HOW YOUR RELATIONSHIP EVOLVES ALONG THE DEMENTIA JOURNEY

Your relationship with your loved one will change along the dementia journey. As detailed in Chapter 1, dementia stages don't have clear boundaries. Some aspects are lost, others are not; but the relationship constantly evolves.

Even before your loved one is diagnosed with dementia, you might start to notice unusual signs. It may be in the form of memory loss and repetition of the same idea, difficulty managing money or medication, disorientation in time and place, language comprehension and expression problems, problem-solving challenges, misplacing everyday objects such as plates or utensils, changes in personality, mood, and behaviors, loss of interest for activities they used to enjoy very much. Once you realize these patterns are repeating themselves, you begin having serious doubts.

When you ask your loved one to carry out routine tasks, only to find they cannot execute them, you may start wondering whether it's simply a result of the natural aging process, or if it's possibly something more. You can enter a state of denial due to this conflicting information, and decide not to look into it further. Statements like, "Mom's just doing this to gain attention," or "She's doing it on purpose," may be in your thoughts as you try to make sense of what you see or hear. You may even say them aloud.

In any case, you must consult a General Practitioner as quickly as possible, as those signs *could* also indicate a curable and more acute condition than dementia, such as delirium. The General Practitioner might refer your loved one to a neurologist if they suspect dementia.

However, as mentioned earlier, getting an official dementia diagnosis can be a very long process because all other possibilities need to be ruled out before concluding whether it is indeed dementia. After weeks, months, or sometimes years of extensive tests, your loved one finally gets an official diagnosis of dementia. And, as we have seen in Chapter 2, after the initial shock of the diagnosis, you may feel lost. You don't understand what's happening, or why. You're starting a journey you didn't ask for, with no information; and you're scared.

So, you begin to look for more information on the internet, watch YouTube videos, read books, and ask people what they know. It may take a while to gain the clarity you need to understand dementia and your part in it. You may be confused about separating the personality of your loved one and their dementia, and that is completely normal. At times, you might even think your loved one with dementia might be faking it or merely using the "excuse" of dementia to trick you into spending more time with them.

Maybe you're afraid, anxious, or frustrated about the changes already happening (and are yet to happen) in your relationship with your loved one. So, next, we'll explore some directions to help you along your journey with your loved one with dementia.

SET GOALS TO EXPERIENCE THE BEST RELATIONSHIP WITH YOUR LOVED ONE WITH DEMENTIA

When stressed, our brains often focus on things that seem threatening. It happens to all of us. As a dementia caregiver, planning or setting goals can be difficult because urgent situations consume your daily life. But don't worry, I'm here to help. I have a step-by-step plan with many valuable tips in the following section. Together, we'll create goals to help you build a strong and loving relationship with your loved one. Even though there will be tough times and challenges ahead, remember that moments of happiness are still very much possible.

TIP #1 TO UNDERSTAND DEMENTIA: LEARN CONTINUOUSLY

Your goal here is to get the maximum amount of valuable information available to understand what the future has in store. It is time to prepare for what comes next. The more you know (especially what *not* to do), the more prepared you will be, and the less likely you will feel lost. Knowledge reduces anxiety levels, even if uncertainty remains. If you understand what you're up against and learn to live with dementia instead of resisting it, you will find even more ways to connect with your loved one.

Tips on what to do if you want to learn continuously

Identify the critical problems you are facing now, get information from professionals/peers/books/videos/programs, etc., and try solutions one step at a time.

- Focus on what you can control, not on what you can't.

- Share what you've learned with family, friends, and professionals; doing so will reinforce the knowledge needed to implement it.
- Be open to new information, new ways of doing things, and new standards of what is suitable for your loved one with dementia.
- Count on the compound effect: a little information and small changes daily will bring tremendous results over time.
- Begin with manageable, tiny changes; it will help build confidence and motivation.
- Adapt your learning curve to the dementia stage your loved one is in.
- Learn to live differently, even if it is far from what you're used to (choose your battles wisely: where will you expend your energy? A harmonious relationship with your loved one with dementia, or your own spiritual, psychological, or physical comfort).
- Share your goals with friends or family who can provide encouragement and hold you accountable.
- Even when you don't feel like it, try your best to smile. Persons with dementia have strong emotional memories. Your loved one may forget who you are and what you did, but not how they felt when you smiled at them.

Tips on what NOT to do if you want to learn continuously

- Do not try to solve every problem so you and your loved one can return to life *before* dementia (as heartbreaking as it is, dementia is a hard truth that needs to be accepted).
- Do not attempt to address every problem at the same time.
- Do not think a professional cannot advise you on strategies to implement with your loved one because you've known him/her longer and understand them better.
- Do not take things personally if a professional tells you to change *your* behaviors if you want to see a change in the behaviors of your loved one with dementia.

- Do not cling to good manners (expecting your loved one with dementia to say "hello", eat properly, bathe every day, and answer when a question is asked); otherwise, you will waste precious energy that could be used elsewhere.

TIP #2 TO ENHANCE WELL-BEING AND ENGAGEMENT: CREATE AN ACTIVITY SCHEDULE

You want to create an activity schedule for your loved one with dementia, which includes a self-care routine for yourself. Build this daily schedule around your loved one with dementia's habits for meals, naps, and sleeping hours.

Consider this as a guide, and not a strict schedule that must be followed by the book. Although consistency is key to forming new habits, the objective here is to set a routine. Here is a simple example to guide you.

HOURS	MON	TUE	WED	THUR	FRI	SAT	SUN
6:30-7:00	Your morning routine for yourself						
7:00-8:00	Your loved one with dementia is waking up: soft music/glass of water/prayer/light stretches/etc...						
8:00-10:00	Breakfast and medication						
10:00-12:30	Adult Daycare program for your loved one	Easy-to-follow recipes (ex: fruit salad)	Shower/Bath (spa day)	Soft gym (ex: chair exercises)	Shower Medical visit or Little walk	Dancing Bingo	Shower Going to church
12:30-14:00		Meal					
14:00-16:00	You the caregiver go to the grocery store/Have rest/Special selfcare moment	Arts and crafts	Laundry with your loved one Sorting socks	Singing Little walk	Laundry with your loved one Arts and crafts	Movie	Arts and crafts
16:00-18:00	Supper and Medication						
18:00-20:00	Dental care, Soft lighting and Gentle massaging before putting on pajamas						
20:00-22:00	Evening routine for you and your loved one (calm voice, relaxing music, reading, praying, etc...)						

TIP #3 TO CREATE A POSITIVE EXPERIENCE DURING MEALTIME: NOURISHING WITH CARE AND COMFORT

Tips on what to do for meals

- Prepare or buy healthy meals for your loved one with dementia. The Mediterranean diet is a good reference.
- Taking medication often matches mealtimes. Ask your loved one's doctor and pharmacist which pill(s) to give at what times, and follow their instructions on how to administer them (for instance: you may have to crush up some pills and mix it with food or a drink to ensure your loved one with dementia takes it).
- Make sure medication is stored in a pill dispenser, out of reach, or locked in a cabinet.
- Use meal delivery services specifically for older adults, such as "Meals on Wheels". Otherwise, you can get frozen and takeout meals. It's not as healthy, but occasionally, it will save you time and effort.
- Practice a quiet activity before a meal.
- Be face-to-face and slowly announce what is on the plate, give short instructions.
- Before eating, allow your loved one to see their food and enjoy the pleasant smells to help stimulate appetite.
- Make sure the food is appropriately sized and limit the variety to three types; give choices.
- Favor food that your loved one with dementia can eat with bare hands instead of utensils, especially if they have apraxia (inability to carry out coordinated movements).
- Make sure the plate or bowl contrasts with the placemat or tablecloth.
- Wait until your loved one with dementia swallows before allowing them to take another bite; and provide one course at a time.
- Use anti-slip mats to put under the plates.

- Make sure your loved one with dementia drinks regularly during the day as they may forget.
- If your loved one with dementia gains or loses a lot of weight, consult a nutritionist.
- Make sure dentures are well-adjusted so your loved one can eat without hurting themselves.
- Verify that your loved one with dementia doesn't hide food. Reassure them that they will have regular snacks throughout the day.
- Have healthy snacks such as raw vegetables ready and visible.
- Because of their medication, your loved one with dementia could have a dry mouth. Make sure you have them drink water while eating.

Tips on what NOT to do for meals

- Avoid unhealthy meals. They trigger many health issues, which worsen dementia behaviors.
- Avoid unnecessary noise/distractions (good lighting and pleasant background sounds – nature/music)
- Don't have dark food on dark plates; your loved one will have difficulty differentiating the food from the container it is served on.
- Don't have patterned tablecloths, placemats or plates. A white plate against a dark background enhance visibility.
- Don't force your loved one with dementia to sit down to eat if they don't want to. But give them tiny pieces of food to eat while walking.
- Do not worry about messiness. Just wait to clean up until after your loved one with dementia is done eating.
- Hide and lock up any items that could be mistaken as food, such as soap, laundry powder, or washing machine pods.
- Don't make assumptions if you notice changes in your loved one with dementia's physical appearance. For instance,

weight loss may be the result of a disease. Take your loved one to the doctor.

Tips on what to do in case of dysphagia (difficulty swallowing)

- Consult a doctor or nutritionist for a professional evaluation and recommendations.
- Soft foods are easier to swallow.
- Make sure your loved one is seated up straight, head slightly forward.
- Wet the mouth of your loved one to address dry mouth symptoms due to medication.
- Offer a sip of water with each bite.
- Mix food with a liquid (water or juice for instance).
- Depending on the severity of dysphagia, you may have to chop meat, use canned fruits, or grind food in a blender.
- Make sure your loved one stays hydrated. One way to hydrate them if they refuse to drink water is to give them water sweets, also called water balls. Lewis Hornby crafted these treats to address his grandmother's hydration challenges during dementia. They resemble traditional candies in taste and texture, but they are sugar-free, are composed of 95% water, and have added electrolytes. You can buy them online at www.jellydrops.us.
- In late-stage dementia, swallowing difficulties may increase. This is known as buccofacial apraxia. To help your loved one, be patient and use special utensils if necessary. Maintain oral hygiene, offer easy-to-eat finger foods, and create a calm meal environment. Encourage independence by letting your loved one use their hands to eat. Use simple communication, monitor their well-being, and consult a professional when needed. Always prioritize your loved one's comfort over their dignity.
- If your loved one with dementia is constipated, there may be several causes, such as eating processed foods, sweets, cakes, and bread in excess. It could also be an adverse effect of

medication. You may want to give your loved one food rich in fiber and psyllium to help fight constipation.
- In late-stage dementia, tube feeding could be considered an option. Still, this practice remains a topic of debate and controversy in the medical community due to the limited evidence of its benefits, ethical concerns regarding patient autonomy, and the potential for complications. Decisions must be individualized, considering your loved one's values and goals. Tube feeding should be discussed with your loved one with dementia as early as possible, so they can make informed decisions.

Tips on what NOT to do in case of dysphagia

- Avoid small, hard snacks, such as: sweets, candy, chewing gum, nuts, and popcorn, because they present a choking hazard.
- Avoid mixed textures in a soup broth, such as whole or chopped vegetables. Instead, use a blender to prepare your soups.
- When you help your seated loved one eat, do NOT do it from a standing position, as this would force them to lift their head to eat, which increases the risk of choking.

If, despite all your efforts, your loved one with dementia still chokes on their food, it is helpful for you to know how to use the Heimlich Maneuver (sometimes called "abdominal thrusts":

1. Circle their waist from behind with your arms.
2. Close one hand to form a fist, with the thumb against their belly. Position your fist between the navel and breastbone.
3. Holding your fist with the other hand, give a swift upward thrust toward their stomach.
4. Adapt your strength to your loved one's girth. Repeat the maneuver. This should allow your loved one to expel the stuck object.

TIP #4 FOR BETTER SLEEP: CREATE A CALMING ENVIRONMENT

Tips on what to do for better sleep

- Favor calm ambiances: silence, low stimulation (e.g. peaceful conversations, no frustrations), dimmed lighting, warm room temperature, soft music, etc.
- You can softly massage body parts like hands, feet, neck, and back.
- Practice aromatherapy (aromatic plant extracts and essential oils to promote relaxation)

Tips on what NOT to do for better sleep

- Avoid stimulants before bedtime (green tea, ginseng, ginkgo biloba).
- Avoid noise and TV (particularly violent or scary content). Put away all screens at least one hour before bedtime.
- Avoid doing too many activities during the day, and adjust to what your loved one with dementia can bear.
- Avoid drinks that excite or add confusion, especially beverages with caffeine, high sugar content, or alcohol.

TIP #5 TO EXPERIENCE A COMFORTING AND SAFE BATHING EXPERIENCE: EMPLOY A GENTLE APPROACH

Among bathing, showering, dental care, hairstyling, and hair removal, bathing is often what triggers catastrophic reactions. You can refer back to Chapter 3 for a reminder about catastrophic reactions.

Tips on what to do for bathing

- To make your loved one with dementia feel comfortable during a bath, prepare the bathroom properly. You should be sweating in the room if it is at the right temperature so your loved one with dementia is not cold when naked. Also, you can play calm music to create a relaxing environment.

- Put towels on the bath chair. Make sure your loved one sees the towel by a color contrast between the towel and the background.
- Dimming the lights can create a more calming atmosphere.
- To make the bath more comfortable, offer it according to your loved one's habits. This could mean picking a specific time, or asking your loved one whether they prefer a shower or bath whenever possible.
- Use choices or redirection if your loved one resists. Try to make their options more appealing. For example, you could ask, "Would you rather follow me now, or after brushing your hair?" or "We'll get a snack after that."
- Using the word "spa" instead of "bath" can help make the experience sound more luxurious and enjoyable. When preparing to get them into the "spa", use the following steps in the same order every time:

1. Apply palm pressure on your loved one's hands with both your hands to warm up and reassure.
2. Make direct eye contact by squatting down.
3. Simulate on yourself how to take off clothes while softly explaining what you are doing.
4. Help your loved one with dementia to take off their clothes except for their underwear

- Instead of forcing your loved one with dementia to remove their underwear, encourage them to do so by wrapping them in a warm, damp towel. This approach will often prompt them to remove their (now) wet underwear and towel altogether, in order to seek comfort. For women, start by taking off the bra, then wash the body while still commenting on what you're doing. For instance, say, "Now, let's put some soap under your arms."

- Wash the folded flesh, including areas below the breasts, armpits, etc.
- After the shower or bath, immediately dry your loved one with warm towels.
- When drying, tap instead of rubbing, and moisturize the skin afterward.
- Before dressing your loved one with dementia, verify the integrity of their skin for pressure sores, ulcers, or rashes.
- Use soft hair tools and handle hair with great gentleness when styling it for your loved one with dementia.
- If your loved one resists taking a bath, you can use the "doctor's orders" to explain why it's essential.
- If bathing becomes difficult, consider giving a sponge bath instead. You can use a damp sponge or washcloth with no-rinse soap as an alternative.
- Protect your back by using the correct equipment and positioning while lifting and lowering your loved one. You can ask an occupational therapist for advice on how to do this safely.
- Use a transfer bench and bath seat to make it easier for your loved one to get in and out of the bathtub. As dementia progresses, the type of equipment needed may change.

Tips on what NOT to do for bathing

- Don't force bathing or showering, especially if you know your loved one with dementia is in pain. If necessary, consult a medical doctor to ask about medication that could help.
- Don't bathe your loved one without preparing them for this moment. Explain to them what is about to happen beforehand.
- Avoid using bubble baths. A bubble bath can make the bathtub slippery and irritate mucous membranes.
- Don't use a fixed showerhead. Instead, use a hand-held showerhead to make it easier for your loved one to see

where the water comes from and help them feel more comfortable during the bath.

- Don't get offended if your loved one accepts healthcare professionals to help them bathe, but not you. Instead, take this as an opportunity for respite, and use the professional services when you can.
- Don't do what your loved one can do for themself. If your loved one with dementia can do some tasks on their own, let them do them. This will help maintain a sense of accomplishment, independence, and control.
- Avoid leaving the skin wet. Leaving the skin wet can lead to chafing and discomfort. To prevent this, thoroughly dry your loved one after a bath. For drying the wet areas of the body, use cornstarch or baking soda instead of talcum powder, as these are cheaper and healthier alternatives.
- Never leave your loved one alone or unattended in the bath, as, statistically, this is where many accidents occur.
- Don't fill the bathtub too high. Filling the bathtub too high can cause your loved one with dementia to panic, as they may feel like they are in the ocean.
- If your loved one with dementia fears loud noises, avoid using hair dryers and electric razors during their bath.
- If your loved one with dementia cannot bear the pain of hair removal or hot wax, it's best to avoid these methods.

TIP #6 TO MAINTAIN ORAL HEALTH: ATTENTIVE DENTAL CARE

Tips on what to do for dental care

- Clean your loved one's teeth or dentures twice a day. Poor oral health can result in chewing and swallowing difficulties, malnutrition, loss of sleep, low self-esteem, decreased ability to communicate, avoidance of social interaction, pain, and increased susceptibility to systemic infectious diseases such as pneumonia

- Ensure that the dentures adhere correctly to your loved one's gums; otherwise, they will face additional challenges while chewing.
- Select a toothbrush with a thickness that allows your loved one with dementia to grip it easily, and choose toothpaste that does not produce excessive foam.
- If your loved one with dementia tends to bite, consider using two toothbrushes as depicted in the following illustration.

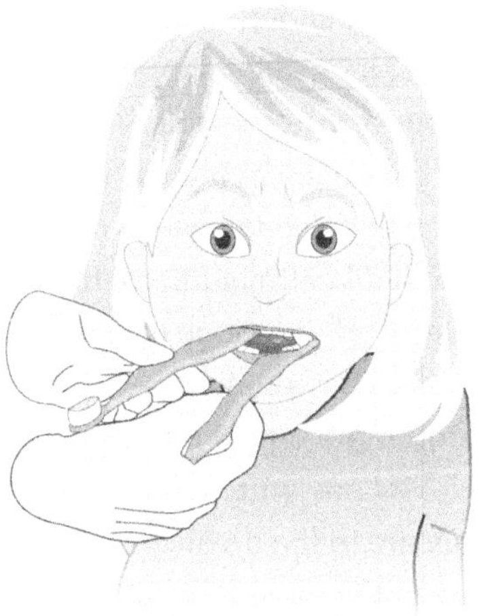

- To encourage independent actions, initiate the movements with your loved one, such as guiding their hand towards their toothbrush and teeth. See if this prompts them to brush their teeth on their own.

Tips on what NOT to do for dental care

- Do not underestimate dental problems and their impact on your loved one's mood. Consult a dentist as soon as possible if you notice something out of the ordinary.

- Do not skip dental care; it is more important than it seems (see 1st dental care bullet point).

TIP #7 TO MANAGE INCONTINENCE WITH DIGNITY: ANTICIPATING NEEDS

Tips on what to do for incontinence

- Consider having an occupational therapist assess your loved one's motor abilities to determine what tasks they can or cannot perform.
- Use urinary incontinence supplies as necessary for your loved one with dementia.
- Urinary tract infections (UTIs) are common among individuals with dementia. Consult a doctor immediately if you observe any signs of a UTI, and report them to a healthcare professional. UTIs can also be related to other conditions, so seeking medical advice is essential.
- To prevent nighttime wetness, limit the amount of water your loved one with dementia drinks before bedtime.
- Have waterproof mattress covers readily available.
- Regularly remind your loved one with dementia to use the bathroom and assist them, if necessary.
- If persistent odors are an issue, utilize baking soda and vinegar while washing their clothes.
- If you find changing briefs unpleasant due to a personal sensitivity to odors or sheer disgust, try these tips to make it more manageable. Create a more positive experience by playing soothing music, or use essential oils to create a pleasant atmosphere while changing your loved one's briefs.
- Wear a mask or use a scented face covering, use disposable gloves, and ensure adequate room ventilation.
- Be efficient during the change, share caregiving tasks if possible, and consider seeking support from professionals or a support group to cope with your feelings.

- Remember to prioritize your well-being as a caregiver, and after changing the soiled briefs, use this time for cuddling or doing some other enjoyable activities with your loved one.

Tips on what NOT to do for incontinence

- Don't criticize your loved one with dementia when they have accidents. Criticism can lead to feelings of shame and discomfort.
- Don't wait to change soiled briefs. Do it as soon as possible to prevent sores from appearing. Make sure your loved one with dementia is always clean and dry.
- Avoid pressuring your loved one to wear briefs. Instead, consider switching from regular underwear to only providing briefs in their closet or dresser drawer.

TIP #8 TO ENHANCE COMFORT AND INDEPENDENCE: THOUGHTFUL CLOTHING

Tips on what to do for clothing

- Simplify the steps for getting dressed by offering easy choices to your loved one with dementia. For example, if they have trouble deciding between two articles of clothing, ask them to choose the color they prefer: blue or yellow.
- When buttons or zippers become difficult for your loved one, opt for clothing with Velcro closures, for convenience.
- Choose loose-fitting clothes that will provide comfort for your loved one with dementia and, at the same time, make it easier for you to assist them when needed.
- Guide your loved one through each step of getting dressed, but choose your battles wisely. If they resist certain clothing choices, allow them to wear what they prefer rather than what you think is more fashionable.
- Consider using satin or silk sheets and pajamas to facilitate movement for your loved one in bed.

Tips on what NOT to do for clothing

- If your loved one with dementia refuses to change clothes, avoid forcing them. Instead, ensure they dress appropriately for the current weather to maintain their comfort and well-being.
- When assisting your loved one with dressing, be cautious to practice safe handling techniques so as not to cause potential injury to yourself.

TIP #9 TO FOSTER JOY AND CONNECTION: SET UP ENGAGING, READY-TO-USE ACTIVITIES

Tips on what to do for setting up ready-to-use activities

- Prepare in advance a music playlist your loved one enjoys, and play recordings of their favorite musicians. Music not only has the power to reconnect your loved one with dementia to significant moments from their past, but it also evokes emotions, promotes movement, and enhances social skills.
- Engage in imaginative storytelling by starting with a word or phrase.
- Gather diversified crafting materials such as images, magazines, drawings, collages, crafting wood, or dough (only if your loved one with dementia does not put it in their mouth) and place them in a box for creative activities.
- Provide simple puzzles for your loved one with dementia to enjoy.
- Involve your loved one with dementia in household chores they can still do, such as folding, cleaning, and laundry. These activities can provide them with a sense of purpose and involvement.
- Encourage activities like pairing socks, folding and sorting towels and sheets, as it can distract your loved one from other stimuli and make them feel helpful.

- Explore cooking activities together, such as mixing, decorating cupcakes, taste-testing, and preparing smoothies.
- Consider purchasing dolls and stuffed animals, including robotic ones. Though more expensive than regular ones, if they are within your budget, they can bring comfort and joy, especially in the mid to late stages of dementia.
- Motivate your loved one with dementia to participate in an adult day care program, where they can socialize in a safe environment and engage in various activities like exercise, games, brain stimulation, music, and bingo.
- Plan visits from friends and family; just remember to keep them brief. Before their visit, inform your guests about your loved one's behaviors and needs related to dementia.
- Design activities based on interests your loved one had before the onset of dementia. For instance, if they used to enjoy playing the piano, consider ways to provide access to a piano if possible (a small, portable one, for instance).

Tips on what NOT to do for setting up ready-to-use activities

- Avoid introducing activities that are too hard or no longer match your loved one's abilities, as this can lead to frustration and upset feelings, potentially causing challenging behaviors.
- Refrain from pushing your loved one to participate in activities when they feel tired, tense, or upset.
- Treat your loved one with dementia respectfully and avoid patronizing or treating them like children.
- Ensure that your loved one is not left bored, as this can accentuate undesired behaviors.
- If you notice that your loved one with dementia is upset about a particular activity, it is best not to insist on doing it.

TIP #10 TO ASSEMBLE YOUR DREAM SUPPORT TEAM: COMMUNICATION AND CLARITY

Harmonize the contact information in your phone, computer, notebook, or whatever fits your style. The relationship with your loved one with dementia, from your perspective, will be better supported when there are people available to contact whom you are confident can help – possibly family, friends, professionals, and support groups. The burden will be too much for one person alone.

Here is a quick list of guidelines to assist you in building the supportive network you desire (you can find more details and tips on building your "dream team" in Chapter 5).

Tips on what to do to build your support dream team

- Ensure your team consists of multiple experts from different fields to provide comprehensive care for your loved one with dementia (even if you only consult them occasionally).
- Seek out professionals with experience or a particular interest in treating dementia, as their expertise can significantly contribute to the care and support provided.
- Strive to establish a trustworthy relationship with healthcare professionals involved in your loved one's care. Building solid rapport can enhance communication and collaboration. Be truthful and transparent about your experiences and feelings.
- Look for professionals who, if not available themselves, can refer you to other qualified individuals for ongoing care and follow-up.
- Clearly define responsibilities and set boundaries, especially when sharing caregiving duties with other family members. This ensures everyone is on the same page and helps avoid misunderstandings.
- Ask questions until you fully understand the information healthcare professionals provide. Clear communication is crucial for making informed decisions and actively participating in the care process.

Tips on what NOT to do to build your support dream team

- Do not disregard the advice and medication that skilled professionals prescribe for your loved one with dementia. Compliance with their recommendations can improve your loved one's overall care and well-being.
- Do not engage in sweeping criticisms about professionals. Instead, when you have concerns or suggestions for improvement related to your loved one's care, focus on specific behaviors or facts that need attention. Be precise in your feedback to promote effective communication.
- Do not resort to harassment or express frustration inappropriately when dealing with professionals. Remember that maintaining a respectful and constructive demeanor is essential for effective communication and collaboration with healthcare providers.

TIP #11 TO ENSURE FINANCIAL SECURITY: ANALYZE YOUR LOVED ONE'S FINANCIAL SUSTAINABILITY

Many caregivers realize their loved one with dementia faces significant challenges when they discover the money is no longer well managed. These problems are often hard to handle alone. Ask for help from your family or a professional. There will most likely be a lot of paperwork to sort through and fill out.

Tips on what to do to analyze your loved one's financial sustainability

- Determine if your loved one is eligible for Medicare or Medicaid, and consider consulting a certified Medicaid planner for guidance on navigating the process.
- Develop a financial plan by assessing your loved one with dementia's financial assets and debts. Create a spreadsheet to record all relevant information. Seek assistance from family, friends, professionals, or associations to complete this assessment.

- Collect passwords, account information, and bills while your loved one with dementia still remembers them. This will help you, or the person who manages your loved one's finances, to oversee them effectively.
- Obtain a power of attorney for accounts, property, and fiduciary matters. Consult a legal advisor experienced in elder law and estate planning. A power of attorney is a legal document that grants someone the authority to make decisions on behalf of another person regarding finances or property if they become incapacitated. The person endowed with this authority is known as a fiduciary.
- Research the cost of care in your region, and assess what you can afford regarding support. Consider assembling a reliable support network (your "dream team"), which may include professionals or organizations that provide affordable or complimentary services.
- Join associations in your region, as they may offer resources, information, and access to low-cost (or no-cost) services to assist you and your loved one with dementia.
- The Association for Financial Counseling and Planning Education (AFCPE.org) can aid a caregiver by providing specialized training and resources related to financial planning and management specific to dementia care. It may include guidance on managing medical costs, setting up a durable power of attorney, understanding insurance, and planning for long-term care.
- Contact your state or local bar association, or visit the National Academy of Elder Law Attorneys (NAELA) website to locate qualified attorneys.
- Ensure that your loved one with dementia has a valid and up-to-date will, ideally created during the early stages of their condition. A will officializes their wishes regarding their assets and estate.
- Contact your loved one's long-term care insurance provider to understand what the policy covers and utilize it accordingly. It's important to note that Medicare and

Medicaid typically do *not* cover long-term care costs for middle-class families.

- Keep all healthcare-related receipts before applying for Medicaid. These receipts can be valuable when applying for Medicaid benefits because they prove your loved one with dementia paid for their own care in the past.
- Share or give financial responsibilities to someone you trust.

Tips on what NOT to do to analyze your loved one's financial sustainability

- Even if you are not comfortable or knowledgeable about financial matters, avoid neglecting the topic of money when caring for your loved one with dementia.
- Don't delay obtaining passwords and establishing power of attorney for your loved one's financial affairs. These steps are crucial for effective management and decision-making when the time comes.
- Refrain from making impulsive purchases that could strain your financial resources. Selflessly consider and plan for your loved one's care expenses instead.
- When determining eligibility for Medicare or Medicaid, avoid making decisions on your own. Seek guidance from professionals or experts who can provide accurate information and assistance in navigating the application process.

TIP #12 TO DEVELOP A DEMENTIA-FRIENDLY AND SAFE HOME ENVIRONMENT: IMPLEMENT ESSENTIAL ADAPTATIONS

Make sure your loved one's environment is dementia-friendly and safe. If you plan to keep your loved one with dementia at home, you must make changes around the house. From the beginning, it will be best to know these upcoming changes and plan for them in advance. Here are a few tips to help you know what to expect.

Tips on what to do to adapt your home and habits for physical safety

- Maintaining a clean and uncluttered home with minimal furniture can significantly reduce the risk of accidents such as falls. This is particularly important if you are caring for a dementia patient who uses assistive devices such as a walker or wheelchair.
- To enhance safety further, you might consider ensuring your flooring is leveled and has no tripping hazards.

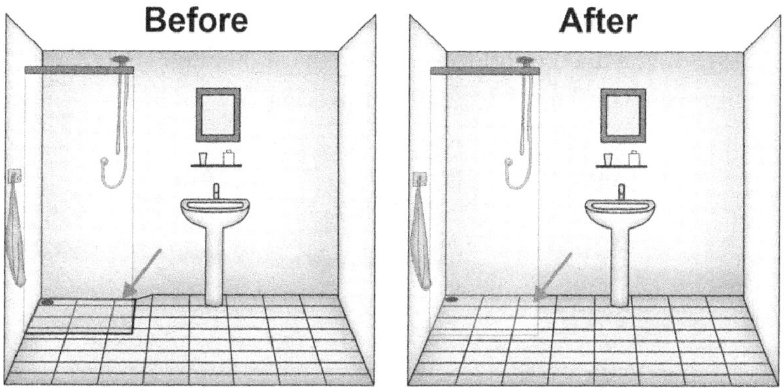

- It is beneficial to install handrails not only in bathrooms and staircases, but also around the bed of your loved one with dementia, if possible. These additional supports can aid in mobility and prevent unexpected falls.

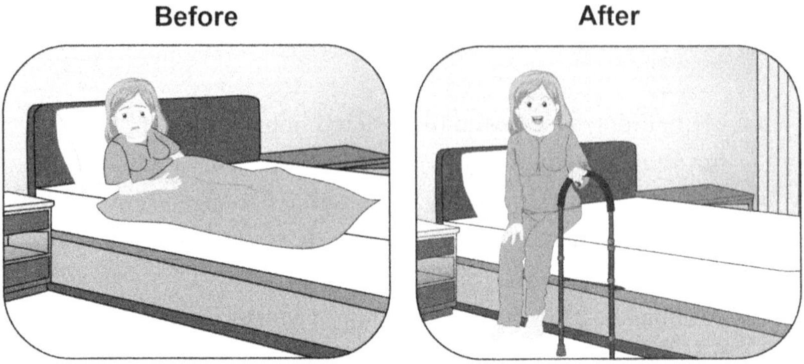

- Modifying your home's water heater to a lower temperature setting can minimize the risk of accidental burns.
- Adding a fixed or foldable seat in the shower will help prevent slips and falls while showering.

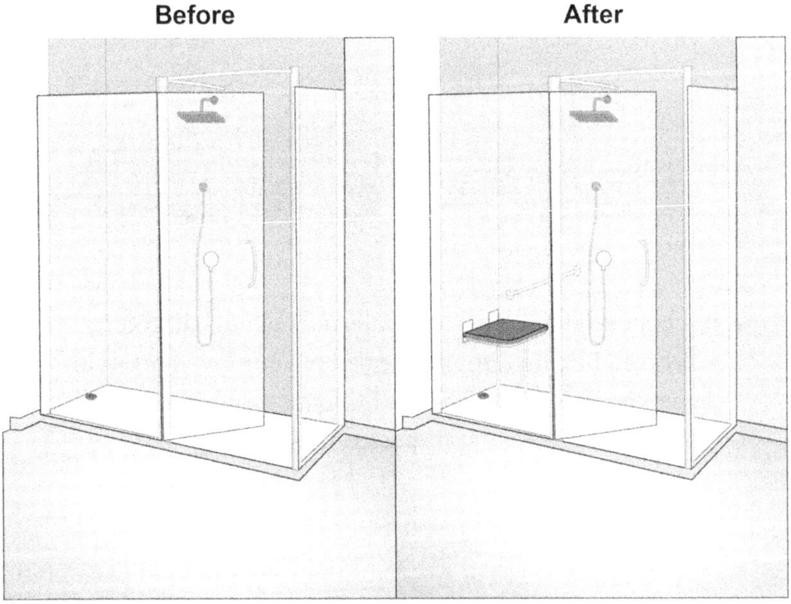

- Utilizing elevated toilet seats and handrails can make the bathroom experience safer and more comfortable for individuals with dementia. It might be worthwhile to inquire with Medicare, or your private insurance provider, to see if they can cover the costs of such adaptive equipment.

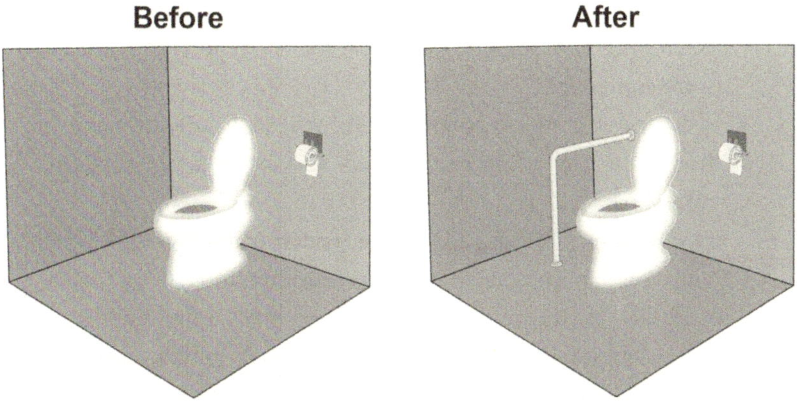

- To prevent your loved one with dementia from accessing unwanted or potentially harmful areas, consider locking some doors or drawers.
- Lock away medications, cleaning substances (shampoo, soap, bleach, etc.), and gardening chemicals.
- Beware of floors that have dark or black-and-white patterns. Such motifs can trigger visual distortions in your loved one's vulnerable brain, leading to confusion and distress. Just imagine the fear they might experience when black tiles appear as treacherous holes in the ground, causing them to freeze up or panic.
- If needed, consider using contrasting colors if your home features a predominantly white interior. Highlighting doors by adding color, either by tape or paint, that contrasts with the white can help your loved one with dementia identify their locations more easily. Even though this might not align with your aesthetic preferences, it could significantly increase the practicality and ease of mobility around your home.
- Conversely, if there are doors you'd prefer your loved one not to notice (such as a laundry room where hazardous

substances are stored), painting the door frames the same color as the walls can help camouflage these areas.

- Placing signs, arrows, and oversized digital clocks on doors or within hallways can provide additional guidance for your loved one with dementia, helping them navigate the house more confidently.
- You can write messages indicating who will care for them during the day while you're gone, and let them know when you'll be back.
- Installing motion sensor lights near stairs and close to their bedroom can improve nighttime visibility and safety, especially if your loved one frequently wakes up at night.
- Consider installing surveillance cameras or baby monitors to allow you to monitor your loved one with dementia, ensuring their safety and well-being.
- If your loved one is at risk of wandering, ensure they wear identification jewelry (necklaces, bracelets, pendants, or rings) that includes contact information.
- Register your loved one with dementia in the "Safe Return Program." This is a nationwide program established by the Alzheimer's Association in collaboration with law enforcement agencies and community organizations. The goal is to help quickly locate and return individuals with dementia who wander and become lost.
- Ensure that the television programming is enjoyable and non-threatening for your loved one with dementia. Avoiding stressful or frightening content can improve your loved one's comfort and well-being.
- To further minimize the risk of falls, consider removing throw rugs and extension cords that could trip up your loved one with dementia.

Tips on what NOT to do to adapt your home and habits for physical safety

- Furniture that is low to the ground or has overly soft cushions can be challenging for your loved one with dementia. Avoid them. Instead, opt for chairs that provide a firm seating surface and are at a comfortable height for both sitting and standing.
- Beware of dark areas in your home. Adding extra lighting fixtures enhances visibility and minimizes shadow plays that might lead to confusion for someone with dementia.
- Limiting access to staircases or minimizing the number of steps within your home can reduce the risk of falls. If there are small steps between rooms, consider installing removable wooden ramps to ease mobility.

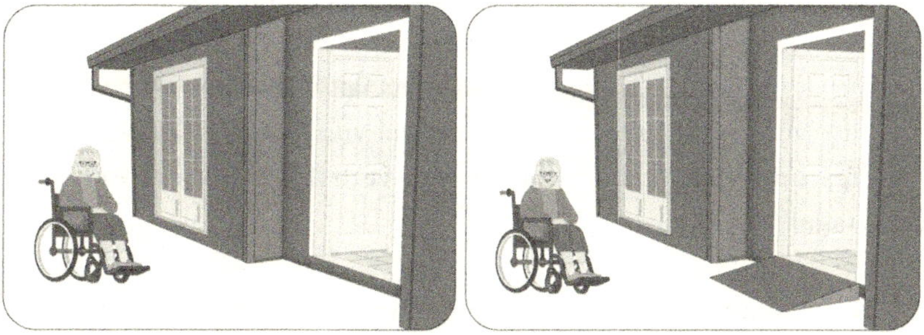

- Restricting access to glassware or other breakable items can prevent accidents and potential injuries.
- If certain decorative items, such as mirrors and paintings, cause distress or confuse your loved one with dementia, it may be best to remove them to reduce the likelihood of disorientation and maintain a calming environment.
- Fire hazards are a common concern when caring for someone with dementia. Therefore, keep items like lighters and matches out of reach. If your loved one is a smoker, always keep an eye on them while they're smoking.

- Consider simplifying your home décor. Patterns can confuse your loved one with dementia, as they may perceive them as tangible objects they can pick up.
- If your loved one with dementia falls, do not let the day pass without getting medical help. Talking to a healthcare professional is necessary even if you can't see any injuries. There could be hidden damage, like a head injury from hitting the floor or a possible bone fracture.

TIP #13 TO ENHANCE COMMUNICATION WITH YOUR LOVED ONE: UTILIZE VERBAL AND NON-VERBAL STRATEGIES

Throughout the dementia journey, keep the humanistic approach in mind. We explored this a little earlier, but the humanistic approach involves fostering a positive caregiving atmosphere by cherishing your loved one's enduring strengths, including non-verbal communication abilities. Your loved one often mirrors your non-verbal cues, so maintaining a peaceful environment is crucial. Here are some tips to enhance your non-verbal communication with them.

Tips on what to do for good non-verbal communication (body language)

- Maintaining eye contact can be a way to effectively connect with your loved one with dementia by conveying attention and understanding.
- Smiling and maintaining positive facial expressions can help create a comforting and cheerful atmosphere, which can be particularly beneficial for someone with dementia.
- Using a calm and soothing voice can help alleviate anxiety or confusion, contributing to more effective communication.
- Gentle touches, hand-holding, and warm hugs can provide a sense of security and reassurance, so long as your loved one with dementia is comfortable with these actions (offering soft touches can provide a tangible sense of comfort and companionship).

- For spouses and partners, prioritize emotional connection through gentle touch when intimacy is no longer well received. Experiencing rejected intimacy can evoke a complex mix of emotions, including sadness, confusion, and a sense of loss for the connection you and your partner with dementia once shared. Look for a therapist to help you navigate this difficult situation.
- Adopting an open posture, and using open-handed arm and hand gestures, can facilitate trust and openness, potentially making your loved one feel more at ease.
- If your loved one with dementia becomes disoriented when they don't see you for a while, consider using a soft alarm to indicate when you'll be back. The sound can serve as a comforting reminder of your imminent return.
- Encourage your loved one with dementia to use non-verbal communication, like pointing at objects, if they struggle with verbal expression. Employing these methods can help them convey their needs more effectively.
- Strategically placed written messages can serve as helpful reminders or guides, provided your loved one with dementia can still comprehend what they are reading.
- Using images or pictograms can be a powerful communication tool, as these visual aids can be easier to understand for someone with dementia.
- Paying close attention to your loved one's non-verbal cues can offer valuable insights into their needs and feelings. These cues can sometimes be more accurate in expressing their meaning than verbal communication.

Tips on what NOT to do for good non-verbal communication (body language)

- Refrain from using an angry tone of voice when communicating with your loved one with dementia. It can be challenging when you're exhausted or hurt by your loved one with dementia's words, but maintaining a calm demeanor is crucial for effective communication.

- Don't steal their personal space and autonomy: Always respect your loved one with dementia's privacy. Be mindful of your loved one's boundaries and avoid uninvited physical contact or intruding on their privacy. This respect can help maintain a sense of dignity and trust.
- Exercise patience and avoid rushing your loved one with dementia, particularly when they're feeling unwell. Hastening their performance may lead to agitation or adverse reactions.
- If your loved one with dementia exhibits aggressive behavior, such as pinching, biting, or kicking, avoid confrontation while ensuring they are safe. Instead, discontinue the activity that may have triggered the aggression and calmly attempt to defuse the situation. Position yourself on their non-dominant side (for example, if they are right-handed, set yourself on their left side), maintain a safe distance, and speak soothingly. Avoid direct eye contact during these times, and provide personal space while offering distractions (try to draw their attention to familiar objects or activities). The goal is to create a non-confrontational environment that reduces their distress. Seek professional assistance or help from other caregivers if the situation becomes unmanageable or unsafe.
- Lastly, if your loved one with dementia can read words but struggles to understand their meaning, practice patience and empathy. Recognize that decoding text and comprehending the meaning are two distinct skills, and cognitive decline may impact your loved one's ability to fully grasp written information.

Tips on what to do for good verbal communication

- Be mindful of potential hearing or vision issues your loved one with dementia may have. Approach them from the side with better hearing or vision, and make your presence known beforehand. If you suspect more severe hearing or sight problems, consider taking them to the doctor for an evaluation.

- Remember to involve your loved one with dementia in any decisions they can make themselves, even if it means going through a trial-and-error process to find the best approach.
- Use respectful language and maintain your composure, even if your loved one with dementia becomes insulting or accusatory.
- Acknowledge your loved one's feelings, and try to redirect them instead of arguing. For example, if they desire to go home, empathize with their emotions, offer comfort with familiar items, and say, "It's already late. We'll stay here for the night, and go home as soon as you wake up." When your loved one is aggressive, acknowledge what they feel by saying, "I'm sorry you feel bad," and try to redirect with, "Let's put on the music you like most."
- Offer choices to your loved one with dementia, allowing them a sense of autonomy and involvement.
- Communicate using brief sentences or questions, and focus on one task at a time.
- Gently suggest alternative activities if your loved one with dementia fixates on repetitive actions. Boredom and anxiety are common triggers.
- Practice patience and reassurance when your loved one with dementia repeats questions or statements, understanding that their need for safety may be driving this behavior.
- Patiently repeat your answers to repeated questions, providing reassurance and stability.
- Speak slowly, leave pauses, and provide short, simple instructions.
- Establish eye contact and smile before continuing with your interaction.
- Use a gentle touch to get your loved one's attention if they have difficulty hearing or seeing you.

- Encourage and praise your loved one with dementia by using positive reinforcement and expressions of appreciation.
- Reassure your loved one by saying, "You are safe. I am with you."
- Set timers for frequent demands, such as medication reminders, to assist your loved one with dementia in adhering to their schedule. Seek help from professionals when needed.
- Offer word suggestions if your loved one with dementia struggles to find the right word. However, use discretion and only continue doing so if you are sure it doesn't upset them. Don't suggest alternatives if they express frustration at your attempts to assist.
- Attempt to acknowledge and appreciate their daily actions, even minor ones: "Good job today." "You did amazing; you deserve a nice rest."
- Ask your loved one with dementia to describe words they're struggling with to help facilitate understanding. For instance, if your loved one says, "I have two trees in my bed," ask them to describe the word "trees."
- Provide reassurance and outline upcoming events when they display anxiety, helping them feel more secure. For instance, you can tell them, "I'll be back in 10 minutes," or "We are going to your favorite grocery store at 9 a.m."
- Foster a sense of respect and autonomy by involving your loved one with dementia as much as possible in daily activities and decision-making.

Tips on what NOT to do for good verbal communication

- Refrain from asking questions that might overwhelm your loved one or lead them to confusion, distress, or frustration. Don't ask *any* questions if your loved one is severely impaired cognitively.

- Avoid speaking negatively about your loved one with dementia in their presence or around others.
- Be respectful and considerate when entering your loved one with dementia's personal space. Give them time to adjust to your presence.
- Avoid discussing sensitive topics, such as toileting or personal clothing, in public areas to preserve your loved one's dignity and privacy.
- If your loved one with dementia experiences an anger outburst, ensure their safety, but consider leaving the immediate area to allow them time to calm down.
- Avoid reminding your loved one with dementia that their condition is the reason for their limitations. Instead, it is better to approach situations empathetically, offering support and encouragement without explicitly linking their struggles to dementia.
- Avoid testing your loved one's memory, as it can cause them distress and potentially create feelings of inadequacy or anger.
- Do not argue, correct, or attempt to reason with your loved one with dementia, as their cognitive decline may limit their ability to understand. Instead, practice active listening, and gently redirect the conversation if needed.
- Do not take things personally. Remember your loved one's behavioral shifts directly result from the underlying physiological alterations in their brain, which can sometimes manifest as criticism towards your food, actions, person, and more.
- Do not give instructions over the phone if your loved one with dementia only understands directives given face-to-face. This practice can ensure more transparent communication and prevent possible confusion.

TIP #14 TO UNLOCK THE BENEFITS OF EXERCISE: ADAPT EVERYDAY PHYSICAL ACTIVITY TO YOUR LOVED ONE'S CONDITION

Exercise offers numerous health benefits for your loved one with dementia, including:

- Reduced risk of falls because of enhanced strength and balance
- Keeping motor skills
- Improved mood
- Better sleep
- Improved memory
- Reduced likelihood of constipation
- Better verbal and non-verbal communication
- Better social skills
- Better behavioral management, such as a decrease in wandering, cursing, and aggressive behavior.

Exercise also helps decrease the frequency and intensity of behavioral and psychological symptoms of dementia while promoting positive interactions.

Here's a guide to start incorporating physical activity into your loved one with dementia's routines.

Tips on what to do to keep your loved one physically active

- Engage your loved one with dementia in enjoyable activities such as dancing, which provides physical exercise, and boosts mood and cognitive engagement.
- Encourage involvement in gardening, an activity that can offer a sense of accomplishment, while also promoting physical movement.
- Allow them to do housework tasks such as vacuuming or folding laundry (under your supervision). This can contribute to maintaining a sense of usefulness and routine.

- Promote walking, an easy, cost-free exercise that helps relieve restlessness and curbs the desire to wander. Consider sheltered locations like malls for walking during inclement weather.
- Utilize a tandem bicycle for cycling activities. Sitting in the front position allows you to have better control of the bike. At the same time, your loved one with dementia enjoys the ride and the outdoor environment.
- Consider chair-based gym exercises, for which you can find instructional videos online. These exercises are great for maintaining muscle strength and flexibility.
- Introduce low-impact aerobics, which you can access via online videos, to provide a gentle yet effective workout.
- To ensure safe outings, have your loved one wear a medical alert bracelet or pendant for an effortless location. Additionally, consider equipping them with a GPS-enabled smartwatch for added tracking convenience.
- If your loved one used to be a fitness guru before dementia, keep up those activities as much as possible. Even if they can't remember all the moves, their muscle memory might surprise you, and bring some joy. I once played table tennis with a dementia patient who was an absolute ninja with the paddle. Whenever he unleashed a sneaky smash that left me dumbfounded, he would burst into laughter, making it clear who the real champ was – and it definitely wasn't me!
- Establish and maintain exercise routines, regularly practicing at the same time. Consistency helps your loved one with dementia adhere to the exercise regimen more easily.
- Always consult a doctor or physical therapist if your loved one with dementia has a specific physical condition like arthritis, apraxia, or osteoporosis to ensure safe and appropriate exercise routines.

Tips on what NOT to do to keep your loved one physically active

- Avoid pushing your loved one to participate in intense physical activities without first consulting a doctor, physiotherapist, or kinesiologist for advice and guidance.
- Do not overwhelm your loved one with dementia by demonstrating numerous movements for them to mimic all at the same time. Instead, guide them through each step individually for better comprehension.
- Before initiating any physical activity, assess your loved one's overall condition, paying attention to potential issues like dizziness, hunger, thirst, sleepiness, or agitation.
- If your loved one with dementia becomes annoyed or upset during an exercise, it's best to halt the activity to avoid further distress.
- If your loved one with dementia falls, don't panic. Reassure them that it will be okay, and place them in the recovery position. Then, call your family doctor or 911, if necessary. However, if your loved one insists on getting up and they seem fine, you can help them up; just be careful not to hurt yourself. Bend your knees with a straight back to lift them. Remember to call your family doctor or a nurse later, even if your loved one appears to be alright now.

TIP #15 TO REDUCE YOUR MENTAL LOAD: BUILD A BACKUP PLAN FOR WHEN YOU CAN NO LONGER PROVIDE CARE

Your ultimate goal throughout your caregiving experience is to find a balance between what your loved one with dementia asks of you and the energy you have to exert in order to meet their essential needs. However, you might be exhausted from long years of caring. You might not recognize yourself anymore, or fail to see the value in your interactions with your loved one. Or, maybe your routine quickly changed because their abilities unexpectedly decreased.

At times like these, it's good to have a backup plan for when you can't handle things on your own anymore. In fact, it would be easier on your future self if you prepared a backup plan *before* it gets to that point. Here are some ways you can start planning ahead.

Tips on what to do to build a backup plan

- Develop a comprehensive plan to safeguard yourself and your loved one with dementia, addressing potential scenarios and solutions.
- Arrange for a reliable substitute caregiver, preferably someone already acquainted with your loved one with dementia, to ensure continuity of care when you are unavailable.
- Don't neglect to provide your substitute with detailed instructions, including emergency contact information, daily routines and schedules, medication guidelines, and strategies for managing the behavioral and psychological symptoms associated with your loved one's dementia.
- Before experiencing caregiver burnout, familiarize yourself with the available resources in your local area. Your loved one with dementia may qualify for affordable, or even free, services. A good starting point is the Alzheimer's Association Community Resource Finder, available at https://www.communityresourcefinder.org/
- Don't hesitate to ask for help from family and friends. Be clear about what kind of assistance you need and graciously accept their help when offered.
- Ensure a legally valid will is in place that reflects the wishes and best interests of your loved one with dementia.
- Foster a transparent and supportive environment by keeping family members informed about the care plans for your loved one with dementia.

Tips on what NOT to do to build a backup plan

- Instead of requesting vague assistance from family and friends (e.g., "I need help"), ask for specific support with clearly defined tasks or time frames (e.g., "On Sundays, between 9:00 a.m. and 2:30 p.m., I need someone to spend time with my loved one with dementia at my home.").

- Rather than discussing the daily routine you've established with your loved one indiscriminately, make an effort to share relevant information in detail with the appropriate people. This will ensure effective communication and collaboration, while at the same time, minimizing ambiguity and misunderstanding.

There are several factors that need to be included when building your backup plan. Let's look at each one a little closer.

Considering Alternate Housing Possibilities

Every long-term care facility follows specific guidelines determining the level of care they can offer. Although these rules can differ by location and facility, having a basic understanding of available care levels will assist you in finding the most suitable care for your loved one.

There is no one-size-fits-all formula for choosing where your loved one with dementia will live because needs change according to the stages of dementia, and each family's situation is unique. But there are generally four combinations from which you can choose.

1. Your loved one with dementia lives alone in a residential setting with paid assistance (in the first stages).
2. Your loved one with dementia lives with you at your home, with either paid assistance or not.
3. Your loved one with dementia lives with you in a residential setting, including medical care and housekeeping.
4. Your loved one with dementia lives alone in a specialized setting with complete care.

Housing options for individuals with dementia in the United States vary depending on the level of care needed, family preferences, and budget. The following list outlines more detailed housing options, along with their pros and cons:

HOUSING OPTION	DEFINITION	MEDICARE, MEDICAID, INSURANCE	PROS	CONS
Long-term care arrangements or Continuing care at home	Services at home which vary from meals to 24/7 services	Medicare: Not typically covered Medicaid: Covered in some cases Insurance: May vary by provider and policy	Staying at home rather than moving.	Admission and monthly fees
Adult Foster Home	The person with dementia lives in a family with someone who provides care	Medicare: Not typically covered Medicaid: Covered in some cases Insurance: May vary by provider and policy	Home-like environment	Rare, costs and quality may vary widely
Domiciliary/ Boarding homes or Personal Care Homes	Homes with supervision for daily living, without complex medical needs	Medicare: Not covered Medicaid: Not covered Insurance: May vary by provider and policy	When specializing in dementia, they generally offer good care.	Dementia specialization is rare, costs and quality may vary widely

HOUSING OPTION	DEFINITION	MEDICARE, MEDICAID, INSURANCE	PROS	CONS
Retirement Housing or Communities, Senior citizen apartments	For individuals in the early stages of Alzheimer's or other forms of dementia who can still independently care for themselves.	Medicare: Not typically covered Medicaid: Covered in some cases Insurance: May vary by provider and policy	Limited supervision (early- onset) and may offer social activities, transportation, and other amenities	Limited supervision
Assisted living facilities or adult living, or residential care communities	Transitional option between independent living and nursing homes.	Medicare: Not typically covered Medicaid: Covered in some cases Insurance: May vary by provider and policy	Housing, meals, supportive services, and healthcare.	Not consistently regulated by the federal government, Services may vary by provider and sate.
Nursing Homes or skilled nursing facilities (SNF)	More intensive medical care for individuals with dementia with complex medical needs. Some have specialized dementia care units.	Medicare: Typically covered Medicaid: Covered in most cases Insurance: May vary by provider and policy	24/7 care, Medical treatment, Nutrition, Care planning, Recreation, Spirituality. Licensed by the state Regulated by the federal government	Varying staff quality and staff-to-resident ratio

HOUSING OPTION	DEFINITION	MEDICARE, MEDICAID, INSURANCE	PROS	CONS
Memory or Alzheimer's Special Care Units (SCUs)	Unit tailored for specific dementia care needs.	Medicare: Typically covered Medicaid: Covered in most cases Insurance: May vary by provider and policy	Specialized care Trained staff	Regulations vary by locations
Life Plan or Life Care Communities or formerly Continuing Care Retirement Communities (CCRCs)	Different levels of care from independent living to nursing home care. Residents can move through these care levels as their needs change.	Medicare: Not typically covered Medicaid: Covered in some cases Insurance: May vary by provider and policy	Flexibility in moving through care levels Continuity of care	Costs vary widely
Hospice Care	Suitable for individuals with advanced dementia and a limited life expectancy. It can provide comfort and support to the individual and their family.	Medicare: Typically covered Medicaid: Covered in most cases Insurance: May vary by provider and policy	Pain management Psychological and/or spiritual care Respite care for caregiver	Limited coverage by insurance Focus on end-of-life

Careful Financial Planning

Whatever choice you make between the four options, be sure to plan accordingly. Some benefits may not be available when taking one option over another. Some options may be associated with a loss of income for your loved one with dementia. For instance, some social security benefits are designed to help elderly persons living alone, and those may stop if your loved one with dementia comes to live in your house. From a tax return perspective, you should be able to declare your loved one with dementia as a dependent living under your roof. Contact a specialized attorney to help you decide your best course of action. If you're not planning on housing your loved one with dementia, you will need to weigh the costs and options of long-term care in your region.

Cost of Long-term Care

To help you plan your budget, let's look at the median costs of long-term care services in 2021, based on the Genworth Cost of Care Survey conducted by *Carescout*. Long-term care services cover home, community-based services, assisted living, and nursing home care.

- Home care: A paid non-medical home health aide's hourly rate is $28, and their weekly rate would be $1,120 (assuming 40 hours of care per week).
- Daycare for adults costs $80 per day.
- Facilities for assisted living: $4,635 per month, or $55,620 annually.
- A private room in a nursing home: $111,657 per year, or $306 per day.
- A semi-private room at a nursing home costs $268 per day, or $97,747 per year.

Moving

Whether you decide to move your loved one or not, challenges are always going to be present, just different. But, to avoid the possibility of their refusing to leave home and move somewhere else, be sure to involve your loved one with dementia in the moving plans. It is also preferable to do this during the early phase (mild dementia), as your loved one will better adapt to their new environment. Generally speaking, moving is already a difficult step. After the transition phase though, things will naturally fall into place. So, don't feel guilty or blame yourself for the decision. Families often wait until their loved one's dementia symptoms become unmanageable at home before considering placing them in a long-term care facility. However, by the time they decide to apply to a long-term care facility, it may be too late, due to waiting lists and administrative procedures causing further delays. As a result, family members sometimes endure extreme emotional turmoil, and struggle to adequately care for their loved ones at home for an extended (and often, indefinite) period of time. Deciding for long-term care for your loved one with dementia is undeniably a challenging affair that adds to your grief. But sometimes, it *is* the best option for your loved one's health and well-being.If you're wondering when your loved one needs long-term care, ask yourself the following questions:

- Do you find assisting your loved one with their hygiene, daily activities, eating, and sleeping to be challenging beyond your ability to handle?
- Do you detect any major risks to your loved one's (or your own) physical or mental health in the home environment?

If the answer to either of these questions is "yes", it is time to apply for a long-term care facility.

TIP #16 TO EVALUATE THE QUALITY OF CARE IN A FACILITY: FOCUS ON OBSERVING THE PEOPLE INSTEAD OF THE ENVIRONMENT

Tips on what to do to evaluate the quality of care in a facility

- When you look for a facility, conduct in-depth research considering reputation, certifications, staff qualifications, and reviews.
- Visit several facilities to assess the environment, cleanliness, safety measures, amenities available for use, and the overall

atmosphere. Observe the way staff members engage with residents.

- Ask for the staff-to-resident ratio and the staff's training related to dementia care, especially behavior management.
- Confirm that the facility has appropriate safety measures, such as alarms, secure entry / exit points, and precautions to prevent wandering.
- Ask for the schedule of recreational activities, and check if they are in place.
- Verify that the facility is licensed, accredited, and compliant with regulatory requirements for dementia care.
- Assess the availability of medical services.
- Clearly understand the costs, what is covered, and the financial implications. Inquire about insurance acceptance and available payment options.
- Seek feedback from current residents and their families about their experiences and satisfaction with the facility's care and services.
- Trust your intuition and observe how you feel during your visits.
- Choose a facility that can cater to the evolving needs of your loved one as their dementia progresses. One offering different levels of care within the same facility would be ideal.
- Please seek advice from healthcare professionals, such as geriatricians or social workers, who may have valuable insights and recommendations based on their experience.
- Carefully review contracts, agreements, and legal aspects to ensure they align with your expectations and protect the rights and well-being of your loved one.

If your loved one already lives in a facility

- Ensure a consistent set of caregivers for your loved one with dementia, as familiar faces can provide comfort and stability.

- If possible, regularly visit your loved one with dementia to maintain strong emotional connections and monitor their well-being.
- To ensure your loved one with dementia stays clean and has their hygiene needs met, make it a routine to check their skin condition regularly.
- When you visit your loved one, request a list of the weekly activities organized for your loved one, if such information is not readily provided.
- Ask for a comprehensive list of your loved one with dementia's medications to stay informed about their medical regimen.
- Inquire if the medical staff has implemented non-pharmacological strategies to manage specific dementia symptoms before resorting to medication (mentioned in slightly more detail back in Chapter 3, under the heading of "Catastrophic Reactions and Aggressions").
- Ask if there have been any incidents or problems with your loved one, and check if they have been sleeping well.
- Make sure your loved one is regularly taken out of their room for varied experiences, to avoid feelings of isolation.
- Inquire about the social interactions your loved one with dementia has, particularly if they share their living space with a roommate.

Tips on what NOT to do to evaluate the quality of care in a facility

- Avoid making a hasty decision without thoroughly researching and visiting multiple facilities. Take your time to ensure you're making the best choice for your loved one.
- Avoid assuming that any care facility can adequately address the unique needs of dementia patients. Choose a facility specifically equipped and experienced in dementia care.

- Avoid overlooking the importance of highly trained staff in dementia care. Ensure the facility has well-trained professionals with expertise in dementia-specific care.
- Avoid being solely influenced by a facility's aesthetics or superficial appearances. The quality of care and staff interactions are paramount.
- Don't disregard the feedback from current residents and their families, even if you don't know them very well. Their past experiences can provide critical insights into the day-to-day operations and quality of care.
- Don't overlook safety features and protocols. Ensure the facility has appropriate safety measures to prevent accidents and manage emergencies.
- Don't overlook hidden costs. Clarify all potential expenses and payment structures to prevent unexpected financial burdens.
- Avoid choosing a facility solely based on convenience or its proximity to your home. Focus on the quality of care and services offered, even if it requires more travel.
- Avoid succumbing to high-pressure sales tactics or emotional manipulation. Base your decision on facts, research, and what's best for your loved one's well-being.
- Avoid signing binding arbitration clauses, which generally limit the ability to sue in court.
- When your loved one already lives in a facility, avoid adopting an aggressive attitude or consistently criticizing the care team. Instead, strive to contribute positively to the collective efforts in caring for your loved one with dementia while still being attentive to the quality of care.

CONSIDERING THE DEMENTIA TERMINAL PHASE

Getting prepared for the separation of death

This is a difficult topic to think about, but it is something that needs to be prepared for. Grief and facing the concept of death can be complicated, and the words we use might never fully capture the depth of these emotions. They are intricately intertwined with the unique path you walk alongside your loved one. As you care for your loved one through the progression of dementia, it is essential to recognize that their journey is unique, just as yours is. No one can fully comprehend the complexity of your experiences, and that's okay. Seek professional guidance and support that caters to your specific needs, and remember, you are not alone in this journey.

Take each step with grace and kindness, and remember to take care of yourself too. Your well-being matters. You are appreciated, and your journey is held with the utmost honor and respect. When approaching death, symptoms of dementia eventually worsen to the point that the person can no longer control their bladder or bowel movements. In the terminal phase of dementia, the extensive damage and dysfunction of brain cells and neural connections are the primary contributors to the observed symptoms. As the condition progresses, the breakdown of neural networks and the accumulation of brain damage lead to severe difficulties with cognition, motor skills, and communication. Several typical indicators of impending death include:

- Extreme fatigue
- Confined to bed
- Diminished consciousness
- Restlessness or agitation
- Emaciated appearance
- Decreased consumption of food and liquids
- Trouble swallowing
- Requiring assistance for all personal needs
- Disorientation regarding time or location
- Difficulty maintaining focus or concentration

Death

When an individual with dementia dies, the primary cause of death usually stems from a separate underlying condition or illness rather than the dementia itself. While dementia may contribute to a person's overall health deterioration, compounding it with these secondary conditions leads to their eventual passing. Examples of such conditions include:

- Infections, such as pneumonia and other related conditions.
- The development of bed sores due to immobility and compromised skin integrity.
- Complications arising from diabetes, which can exacerbate overall health issues.
- The presence of heart-kidney disease, where the interaction between heart and kidney dysfunction plays a critical role in the individual's decline.

Grieving

After the passing of your loved one with dementia, although their physical presence is no longer there, the bond you shared remains strong due to the journey you both traversed together. Their habits and memories still linger, reminding you of the precious moments you cherished. It might be challenging to adjust to a life without caregiving responsibilities, as you had previously devoted so much of yourself to their care. Now, you find yourself experiencing a second wave of grief, similar to the one you faced when witnessing the changes in your loved one's personality throughout their dementia journey. In these moments of profound emotions, spirituality can be a guiding light, offering comfort and reassurance. It's essential to prioritize self-care, taking each day one step at a time. Allow yourself the space to grieve, pause, cry, and express any feelings of guilt, sorrow, or emotional wounds that arise. Embrace the spiritual support that surrounds you, finding strength in your faith or religious practice as you navigate through this period of healing and growth. Seek support from friends, family, or professionals who can lend a compassionate ear. When you feel ready, sharing your experience can help you feel better, and bring comfort and understanding to others facing similar situations.

Remember, healing takes time, and feeling a mix of emotions is okay. Embrace the memories and the love you shared with your loved one as you navigate through this period of grief, knowing that you are not alone in your journey of healing and growth.

CHAPTER 5
BUILDING YOUR DREAM TEAM

"*It is not how much you do, but how much love you put into doing.*"
– Mother Teresa

Jennifer had seen firsthand the level of emotional distress dementia was capable of causing her mom. After the experiences she had taking care of her mother, Jennifer couldn't help but come to an understanding about having a nurse come and visit the home. It was a difficult decision financially; but Jennifer knew it was the right thing to do. Since the time Lovely had been diagnosed with dementia, she had needed constant care and supervision. Jennifer knew she couldn't do it all alone. Therefore, it was a perfect time to bring in professional help.

After much deliberation and research, Jennifer hired a care nurse to visit her mother at home. She believed the nurse would monitor her mother's medication, offer assistance when necessary, and provide Lovely the care and emotional support she would require, while allowing Jennifer to take a break. But the nurse did so much more than expected.

The day they met, the nurse introduced Jennifer to the idea of music therapy. She told Jennifer how music could evoke memories and emotions, and that music therapy was a powerful tool that could help reduce Lovely's anxiety, depression, and agitation.

Feeling excited about this new prospect, Jennifer decided to incorporate music therapy sessions to help her mom cope, and started looking for a music therapist who could work with her mother. She searched the Certification Board for Music Therapy (CBMT) website, and found one available.

Watching her mother's face light up at the first session, she knew she had made the right decision. The music therapist led the session through different activities, such as singing, dancing, and playing instruments. Her mother sang along to the songs, clapping her hands, and smiling joyfully. As time passed, she noticed that the sessions developed a positive environment for interaction between herself and her mom, since they both loved music. In addition, her mom sometimes remembered details from a previous session, which was almost nonexistent in other contexts. The music stimulated her mom's emotional memory. Discovering the power music could have on memory and emotions was a small revolution for Jennifer.

Lovely's music therapist also worked for an adult daycare center. Jennifer applied for a spot there through her mother's social worker, and Lovely was accepted a few months later.

During the week, Jennifer would take her mom to the daycare center, and was consistently amazed at the positive changes she saw in her mom. Lovely seemed more relaxed, less agitated, and more connected to her environment. Jennifer soon discovered other professionals at the day center who had experience with dementia, such as an occupational therapist, a speech therapist, and a physical therapist. Her "dream team" was growing exponentially from the useful advice of a single, caring nurse.

Jennifer's decision to employ a care nurse and attend music therapy sessions were some of the best decisions she could have made for her loved one with dementia. She was happy to see her mom smiling and laughing again. She knew she couldn't have done it alone; she learned the importance of teamwork! Jennifer was beyond grateful to have such valuable additions to her circle.

In this chapter, we will help you get to that point in your journey. We'll look at the different healthcare professionals, what they do, and how to build a constructive partnership with them to enable you to assemble your dream team.

PROFESSIONS AROUND DEMENTIA

There are more than ten different healthcare professions associated with dementia. You will most likely encounter experts in various settings, especially at hospitals, as some will be doctors and others nurses. They frequently collaborate with allied health experts like occupational therapists, speech pathologists, and social care providers like social workers.

If your loved one has been recently diagnosed with dementia, they will probably be able to consult various health and social care specialists themselves, or may perhaps need you (the caregiver) to accompany them. Some dementia caregivers may find it a bit hasty and possibly unnecessary this early on, but these specialists offer vital support. They can assist your loved one in living their best life with dementia as soon as possible.

HIRING A HEALTHCARE PROFESSIONAL

When hiring a healthcare professional for your loved one with dementia, consider these essential points to help you make informed decisions:

1. Get references and check licenses and accreditations.
2. Create a file with detailed medical information about your loved one.
3. Keep a journal of any observed changes in your loved one's behavior.
4. In preparation for your call, jot down questions you may have for the professional in your journal.
5. When contacting the professional, ask about their experience, availability, fees, and credentials.

6. Switch professionals if you're unsatisfied with the services provided.
7. If you hire home-care personnel, keep valuable items and medications hidden to prevent theft.
8. Take time to understand your loved one's feelings. If they seem upset or uneasy in the presence of the professional, investigate carefully to ensure their well-being and safety.

YOUR DREAM TEAM

Not all professionals are needed in your dementia caregiving journey. Your dream team will necessarily involve a primary doctor, neurologist or neuropsychologist, a nurse, a pharmacist, a social worker, one or more types of therapists, and an attorney. This basic team will be around you and your loved one in varying capacities. Ideally, though challenging to implement with the current shortage of healthcare workers, keeping the same dream team during your entire caregiving journey would be preferable, as it provides more stability and familiarity. On top of that, you save yourself time and energy because you won't have to constantly repeat instructions or manage a complex schedule.

You, as the caregiver, will play a key role in letting your dream team know about your loved one with dementia's health, preferences, medical history, and recent behavior changes. For effective communication with healthcare professionals, provide precise descriptions of observed behaviors. Consider recording a video to visually demonstrate what you have been witnessing.

Other professionals are likely to be considered for your dream team as they have different expertise and problem-solving skills, but you want to ensure that everyone in your dream team is well-balanced between their professional and human relations skills. Also, make sure the professionals have been adequately trained, and that they have all the credentials required to help your loved one with dementia and also you, as a new caregiver. Ensure their reputation is clean, and no one has filed any complaints against them in the past.

Now, let's explore a little further to learn more about these healthcare professionals and understand how each profession can help you and your loved one with dementia.

1. MEDICAL SPECIALISTS

Promoting health and preventing disease are significant components of your loved one's care. Medical specialists help with this by identifying and treating diseases with medications, diet, and lifestyle changes. If they are unable to do so, they will give referrals.

Primary care doctors, geriatricians, neurologists, and geriatric psychiatrists are the medical specialists who will most likely provide a formal diagnosis for your loved one with dementia. They may evaluate your loved one's life expectancy from a few months to a decade or more, depending on their age, overall health, and type of dementia. They will also be actively involved in the treatment of your loved one with dementia.

Let's further explore the role of each one in the following section.

PRIMARY CARE DOCTORS

Primary care doctors, also known as family care doctors or general practitioners, specialize in general medicine. They are usually the first healthcare professionals you'll see. They can provide comprehensive care for individuals with dementia throughout all stages because they have a deep and long-term understanding of the patient's and their family's medical, social, and emotional needs.

Apart from being the first point of contact for dementia care, they are an essential resource for the early detection of dementia. Patients often consult family care doctors and general practitioners interchangeably, but there are some differences that set them apart. Family doctors prioritize comprehensive care for the entire family, offering health maintenance services for patients across various age groups, from newborns to seniors. Their role as general practitioners involves conducting routine checkups and treating a wide range of medical conditions for individuals of all ages.

A general practitioner serves as a primary care doctor too. Like family medicine physicians, they handle everyday health problems and concentrate on preventing illnesses. They can order diagnostic tests if needed after assessing a medical condition. Your loved one's primary care physician should be the first point of contact regarding general health concerns.

When to consult a primary care doctor?

Before diagnosis, as soon as you notice any signs of cognitive decline in your loved one—changes in their mood, memory, or behaviors—and periodically afterward, involve the general practitioner to monitor their progress and get them on the proper medications.

What to ask a primary care doctor?

As soon as you successfully make contact with a primary care doctor, here are some inquiries you should make to ensure you're not going back and forth in search of primary care doctors:

- Considering the symptoms, do you think my loved one has dementia?
- How familiar are you with diagnosing dementia?
- Do you have good references?
- Should I consider seeing a neurologist?
- Do I have to look for test appointments?
- What can my loved one expect in the upcoming weeks? Months? Years?
- Which care resources are available for my loved one, now and in the future?
- How often does my loved one have to see you?
- When is the next appointment?
- How can I reach you if I have questions or emergencies between appointments?
- I have noticed my loved one has been more confused over the past days: Could it be a urinary tract infection (UTI)?
- What treatment is available?
- What are the risks and benefits of the treatment?
- What resources are available in the community to help?
- Are there any experimental drug trials to participate in?
- Do you give referrals to any other health professionals?

- Can we talk separately after the appointment to share concerns or information without making my loved one anxious?

Asking and getting answers to these questions will assist you in making decisions as time progresses.

Where to find a primary care doctor?

Primary care doctors can be found in various locations:

- Clinics
- Local hospitals
- Long-term care facilities
- Private practices
- Outpatient and inpatient hospital settings
- Group or family practices
- Local Alzheimer's Association
- Dementia Service Association

How to partner with a primary care doctor?

- Prepare for the appointment: make a list of your loved one's symptoms and provide their frequency and duration.
- Prioritize the health issues that impact your loved one's daily life the most. Do not try to cover everything in one single consultation. Book a second appointment if need be.
- Be honest about your loved one's habits, lifestyle, and interactions. The consultation is confidential.
- Encourage your loved one with dementia to follow their care plan. If medications are ineffective or cause major adverse effects, communicate with the doctor for adjustments.
- Support your loved one in understanding their care plan, and following up with further appointments.

GERIATRICIANS

A geriatrician is also a primary care doctor, but they specialize in treating, diagnosing, and preventing diseases and disabilities in older adults. They are more experienced with dementia than regular doctors. They are trained to manage multiple medical conditions related to aging, coordinate care with other health providers, create care plans and set care priorities, evaluate pharmacological treatments, and change medication or dosages if needed. Geriatricians are helpful in many aspects of dementia care, including managing symptoms through medication and evaluating side effects. They generally dedicate more time than other doctors to older adults with dementia.

When to consult a geriatrician?

Dementia is a complex and often age-related condition; therefore, you should consult a geriatrician when you notice the early symptoms of dementia in your loved one; they can help to expose their problems.

What to ask a geriatrician?

Here are a few questions you can ask a geriatrician to get the conversation started:

- Will you replace my loved one's primary care physician? This question ultimately comes down to making your own decision. But if your primary care doctor treats your whole family, and you have developed a relationship over the years, switching might be problematic. However, dementia is a complex condition, and geriatricians are specifically trained to handle and guide you through this kind of complexity.
- Which stage is my loved one in?
- What can I do to help my loved one?

Where to find a geriatrician?

Geriatricians work in acute care hospitals, memory clinics, private practices, community clinics, and residential care. You can use the American Geriatric Society's search tool to find a geriatrician in your area. Still, you should know that finding one will become increasingly more difficult, primarily due to the growth in the aging population, and a shortage of medical professionals who specialize in senior care.

How to partner with a geriatrician?

- Have your loved one's medicine list with you. Make it easy to read. You can bring all your medicines in one bag so the geriatrician can take a look (ask if that would be necessary before the consultation).
- Answer the geriatrician's questions regarding your loved one accurately, but as concisely as possible, to respect their time. Report observable facts regarding your loved one with dementia's behaviors, not your own feelings or fears about what you have witnessed.
- Prepare and organize your questions in advance based on your observations.

NEUROLOGISTS

A neurologist is a doctor who specializes in diagnosing, treating, and managing illnesses related to the brain and nervous system. They are frequently consulted to make dementia diagnoses because they are experts on the subject, and are specifically trained in Alzheimer's and other types of dementia.

Neurologists perform memory evaluations and interpret them based on their extensive knowledge of the brain. Their role is to rule out other underlying conditions potentially related to cognitive decline, and to isolate dementia as the only possible cause. And, since no single diagnostic test can determine if a person is exposed to dementia, neurologists use a variety of approaches to help make a diagnosis. Some of these approaches might be:

- Cognitive tests: Mini-Mental State Exam (MMSE) and Mini-Cog test.
- Neurological tests: Reflexes, muscle tone, eye movement, speech, sensation, and brain imaging.

When to consult a neurologist?

Your family doctor might refer your loved one to a neurologist if they find out after their initial assessment that the symptoms require further investigation. Oftentimes, these referrals aim to get a neurologist involved in the early stages of dementia, even before the symptoms impact your loved one's daily life.

What to ask a neurologist?

During the first visit with a neurologist, you may want some or all of the following questions answered to be fully informed about your loved one's health:

- What is causing my loved one's memory loss?
- What type of dementia does my loved one have?
- How fast does dementia progress, and how long will my loved one live?
- Are there any other functions of the brain possibly affected at this moment?
- How much can my loved one remember at this point?
- What can I do to maintain my loved one's memory and other brain functions for as long as possible?

Where to find a neurologist?

You can ask your primary care doctor for a referral, or contact the neurology department of the medical centers near you. Also, given that neurologists involved in dementia research are often at the forefront of their domain, you can look in the National Institutes of Health's database for ongoing research related to dementia.

How to partner with a neurologist?

- Be honest while describing your loved one's health changes with as many details as possible: memory loss, behavior changes, increased mood swings, etc.
- Bring a list of past and recurrent problems, along with any family history related to these problems.
- A list of all the medicines your loved one currently takes. You can bring them directly in a bag if it's easier for you.

- Have all your questions prepared and written down in advance, to save time and avoid missing anything important.
- Answer the neurologist's questions honestly, with as much accuracy as possible.

GERIATRIC PSYCHIATRISTS

Geriatric psychiatrists, also known as geropsychiatrists, can be an invaluable addition to the devoted team of healthcare professionals caring for your loved one with dementia. These specialists undergo additional training (1 to 2 years) beyond general psychiatry to cater to the distinct needs of older adults, including individuals with dementia. Geriatric psychiatrists bring expertise in managing both physiological and emotional symptoms of dementia and often collaborate closely with neurologists.

Geriatric psychiatrists assess, treat, and prescribe medication to address symptoms shared between some mental health conditions and dementia. Medicare may cover the cost of a psychiatric evaluation and depression screening under certain conditions. A yearly wellness visit, as well as an annual psychiatric assessment, are also usually covered. Seek support and information through the American Association for Geriatric Psychiatry's online search tool at www.aagponline.org or seek a referral from your general practitioner.

When to consult a geriatric psychiatrist?

It's advisable to schedule an appointment with a geriatric psychiatrist for your loved one with dementia if you observe symptoms like delusions, disorientation, hallucinations, aggression, excitement, depression, refusal to eat or drink, or if they start presenting endangering behaviors for themselves or others.

That's another great thing about geriatric psychiatrists, they also offer guidance and support to dementia caregivers like you, who may be dealing with the emotional challenges of caring for someone with dementia. Don't be afraid to address your stress as a caregiver with them, as this significantly impacts how you care for your loved one with dementia. Beyond symptom management, geriatric psychiatrists can also empower you with knowledge. Being well-informed about dementia enhances your ability to cope with stress, ultimately improving the quality of care provided to your loved one with dementia. It's a mutually beneficial arrangement for all parties involved in dementia care.

What to ask a geriatric psychiatrist?

- Can you tell me about my loved one's dementia diagnosis, and its most common symptoms?
- What treatments are available to treat these symptoms and what are the potential benefits and drawbacks of each?
- Which specific medications do you recommend to delay cognitive decline, and manage the behavioral and psychological symptoms of dementia?
- What changes should we make in my loved one's environment, nutrition, and activities to promote physical and mental wellness?
- Do you have recommendations for managing sleep disturbances in my loved one with dementia, and are there specific strategies or interventions that can be employed to improve their sleep patterns?
- Can you suggest a daily routine and activities to minimize the following symptoms… (choose the symptoms that apply the most to your loved one with dementia: anxiety, depression, or agitation, etc.)?
- Can you suggest ways to effectively communicate with my loved one?

Where to find a geriatric psychiatrist?

Ask your primary care doctor or neurologist to refer you to one. Otherwise, consult the American Association for Geriatric Psychiatry's directory: Go to aagponline.org, and in the "Psychiatrists and Providers" tab, select "find a geriatric psychiatrist."

How to partner with a geriatric psychiatrist?

Be as factual as possible in describing your loved one's symptoms, and thoroughly describe your loved one's behaviors at home. Describe how your loved one with dementia was before the onset of dementia to help the geriatric psychiatrist differentiate behaviors related to dementia from those related to your loved one's personality. Keep records of your loved one's appointments with other professionals, such as neurologists, in case communication between the psychiatrist and other professionals is not optimal. If you have trouble finding a geriatric psychiatrist for your loved one with dementia, you may want to consult a general psychiatrist instead. For more information regarding this specialty applied to dementia care, refer to the appendix.

2. CARE AND SUPPORT PROFESSIONALS

DEMENTIA NURSE

Three main types of nurses typically care for people with dementia: Licensed Practical Nurses (LPNs), Registered Nurses (RNs), and Nurse Practitioners (NPs).

Licensed Practical Nurses are the least educated among these three types of nurses. They generally hold a certificate or diploma in practical nursing and have completed a shorter degree. Licensed practical nurses handle fundamental nursing tasks such as taking vital signs, assisting patients with dressing and bathing, and providing essential bedside care. A doctor or registered nurse supervises them.

Registered nurses have completed a more comprehensive curriculum and gained more practical experience than licensed practical nurses. They usually hold a bachelor's degree or a two-year associate's degree in nursing. They can carry out more patient care tasks, such as prescribing specific drugs, running diagnostic tests, and creating care plans. Operating across multiple healthcare settings—ranging from hospitals and nursing homes to community outreach and home-based services—registered nurses play a pivotal role in orchestrating and supervising comprehensive care for individuals. Registered nurses also organize and coordinate the care provided by medical and assistive care personnel. Advanced training in dementia care enables specific registered nurses to assume specialized roles like dementia clinical nurse consultants, nurse practitioners, and dementia nurse advisers.

Finally, nurse practitioners (NPs) are the most qualified nurses in dementia care. They are usually decisive in managing symptoms associated with advanced dementia. In fact, they have further clinical assessment training and can write prescriptions. In addition, their education and in-practice training makes them particularly fit to build and manage the team of professionals around your loved one while still being remarkably attentive to details.

Because the number of nurse practitioners is already significant and growing, Medicare incentivizes caregivers to hire them as leading providers in dementia care instead of medical doctors (MDs). In long-term care facilities, nurse practitioners will likely be your loved one with dementia's leading service providers. Depending on their education and in-practice training, a nurse can offer the following services:

- Develop a good knowledge of your loved one with dementia's life story, and maintain a close relationship with them.
- Provide your loved one with emotional support.
- Manage your loved one's primary care and medication.
- Help you and your loved one with dementia navigate comorbid conditions and polypharmacy (taking several medications at the same time).
- Assess the capacity of your loved one with dementia to make decisions.
- Manage dementia behaviors efficiently.
- Educate other professional staff members and family caregivers.
- They can also verify and encourage your loved one with dementia on: food and fluid intake and physical activities such as, the ability to use the toilet independently.

When to hire a dementia nurse?

Do you need help coordinating care and medication for your loved one with dementia and require an ongoing assessment of their autonomy? If so, you will need the services of a dementia care nurse. The frequency of visits may vary depending on your loved one's healthcare needs, but Medicare covers most home healthcare services. Without Medicare though, the rate for a private, skilled nurse to visit your home varies widely. Depending on your location, rates start around $100 per visit.

If you are in the US, not only do those variations apply between states, but also between cities within the same state. The following link can help you estimate the hourly, monthly, or yearly cost for dementia home care services in your area https://www.genworth.com/aging-and-you/finances/cost-of-care.html.

But just to give you an idea, we will use California as an example (mainly because it has the highest number of Americans aged 65 and older with Alzheimer's dementia). A skilled nursing visit in the Bay Area costs between $55 for independent qualified nurses, and $165 per hour for home care organizations. With inflation in 2022, the rates of some of these organizations went up to $180 per hour.

What to ask a dementia nurse?

If you get one-on-one time with a dementia nurse, here are a few questions you can ask to get started:

- How do you navigate complex care situations with dementia care personnel?
- Can you give me references for local agencies or online resources?
- Can you explain this medication and its side effects?
- Can you give me strategies to give medication to my loved one with dementia, especially if they resist or refuse it?
- Can you help me understand my loved one's behavior changes?
- Can you help me assess if my loved one with dementia feels pain?

Where to find a dementia care nurse?

To find a dementia care nurse that's right for you and your loved one with dementia, you can use the elder care locator at https://eldercare.acl.gov/Public/Index.aspx

How to partner with a dementia nurse?

The idea is to establish a trusting, long-term relationship with them, so look for qualities such as empathy, compassion, clinical experience, sensitivity, dedication, and skills at communicating instructions. Do your best to keep the same nurse for stability around your loved one with dementia.

PHARMACIST

A pharmacist is a healthcare professional specializing in safely and effectively using medications. He or she:

- Can address questions and concerns related to dementia.
- Can offer education about dementia
- Has knowledge of predisposing conditions to dementia, and is more likely to monitor them closely.
- Can provide expert advice for medication to address dementia comorbidities (e.g., urinary tract infection, depression, psychosis, etc.), and can also provide advice on the side effects of medications.
- After a diagnosis of dementia, a pharmacist can help by not blaming dementia for everything, and can still spot symptoms unrelated to dementia (e.g., delirium).

When to consult a pharmacist?

If you observe some of the symptoms of dementia that we discussed in Chapter 1, engaging in a conversation with a pharmacist could be beneficial. They may be familiar with behaviors associated with dementia and should be consulted if you have doubts. Medicare may cover expenses for most (if not all of) the medication they prescribe.

What to ask a pharmacist?

When you have a one-on-one session, here are a few questions you can ask a pharmacist to get the conversation started:

- Should my loved one with dementia stop taking this medication?
- Does this medication help my loved one with dementia?
- Should the dosage be increased/decreased for this medication?
- What side effects should I expect from this medication?

Where to find a pharmacist?

To find a senior care pharmacist, refer to https://www.ascp.com/page/whatisacp and scroll down to the section "ASCP Membership Practice Settings."

How to partner with a pharmacist

- Be curious about medication.
- Target a skilled dementia care pharmacist and build a relationship.

A good pharmacist is knowledgeable, caring, compassionate, attentive, precise, accurate, and friendly.

REGISTERED DIETITIANS (OR OTHER NUTRITION PROFESSIONALS)

Registered dietitians (RDs) are medical practitioners who work with patients with medical disorders that can benefit from dietary intervention, such as diabetes and heart disease. They create nutritional care plans to match the individual's medical conditions and dietary restrictions. The RD may collaborate with speech pathologists and nurses to plan an adequate diet. On the other hand, since registered dietitians specialize in various aspects of nutrition, such as community health and public health nutrition, they may also provide nutrition advice to groups.

In dementia care, RDs develop plans to maintain physical and cognitive health for as long as possible. They also contribute to decreasing behavioral and psychological symptoms of dementia because nutrition directly impacts both.

Dementia patients may have nutritional deficiencies, or start finding it difficult to eat or swallow meals. They might experience weight loss as they progress through the stages. A registered dietitian can provide evidence-based data on the impacts of food and recommend dietary supplements or food intake strategies to overcome these hurdles. Finally, RDs can give caregivers recommendations on meal preparation and feeding techniques for their loved ones with dementia.

When to consult a registered dietitian?

When you start observing changes in your loved one's appetite, swallowing difficulties, or weight loss, it is time to consult a registered dietitian or medical nutrition professional. Other reasons to consult an RD include gastrointestinal problems or other medical conditions affecting their nutritional needs. If you are unsure whether your loved one has been eating properly, trust your instincts and consult a registered dietitian.

What to ask a registered dietitian?

Here are a few questions to ask when consulting an RD:

- Which types of food should be part of my loved one's meal plan? What should they avoid?
- What can I do if my loved one refuses to eat?
- How can I prevent significant weight variations (loss or gain) for my loved one with dementia?
- How can I make my loved one's meal time more enjoyable?
- Which finger foods are good for my loved one with dementia?
- Can certain supplements or vitamins benefit my loved one with dementia?

Where to find a registered dietitian?

Consult the Academy of Nutrition and Dietetics website to locate an RD nearby. Browsing their online directory at www.eatright.org/find-a-nutrition-expert is the most effective way to find one. You can filter results by zip code. Otherwise, seek a referral from your loved one's general practitioner, social worker, or geriatrician.

There is a difference between a registered dietitian and a "nutritionist" (or any other nutrition professional) in the United States. The registered dietitian is always certified by the Academy of Nutrition and Dietetics. In contrast, other nutrition professionals are not necessarily accredited. The Board for Certification of Nutrition Specialists can license nutritionists, however, some states do not require licensure to open a nutrition practice. The RD title guarantees that the professional you consult for your loved one with dementia has, at the very least, completed a Bachelor's degree, a supervised dietetic internship, and has successfully passed a national registration exam.

For individuals with dementia, Medicare Part B typically does not cover medical nutrition therapy services. Those services are covered only for individuals with diabetes and kidney disease, and only if provided by a registered dietitian or nutrition professional with specific qualifications. Conversely, Medicaid may cover nutrition services, including medical nutrition therapy, for individuals with dementia who are eligible for the program. Coverage varies by state, so it's best to check with your state's Medicaid agency to see what nutrition services are covered.

How to partner with a registered dietitian?

Provide factual and exhaustive information about your loved one's medical history, medications, and dietary restrictions. Report any changes in their appetite. Be proactive in developing your loved one's meal plan with the dietitian.

OCCUPATIONAL THERAPIST

Occupational therapists assess clients' functional abilities to care for themselves. Collaborating with clients and caregivers, these health experts aim to optimize freedom and safety at home and in the community. They are involved in cognitive testing, risk assessment, safety issues, task breakdown, equipment guidance, and environmental adaptations to retain independence.

Through the therapeutic use of routine activities, occupational therapists assist people of all ages in participating in the activities they desire and need to do (occupations). They help individuals with ailments affecting their capacity to carry out daily chores, such as physical or developmental limitations, wounds, or chronic illnesses.

Occupational therapists can evaluate your loved one's driving ability, by observing indicators like vision, reaction time, and hearing. When trying to convince your loved one with dementia to stop driving becomes too much of a challenge for you personally, involving experts can be a crucial step. Caregivers could face significant legal and financial trouble if an accident occurs after a doctor recommends discontinuing driving. If you anticipate a risk that your loved one might still drive despite being forbidden, selling the vehicle might be the ultimate solution.

When to consult an occupational therapist?

Consult an occupational therapist if your loved one starts experiencing difficulties performing daily activities. Medicare generally covers 80% of costs when a physician prescribes occupational therapy.

What to ask an occupational therapist?

During your session with an occupational therapist, consider asking the following questions:

- Can you help me set up a routine with my loved one with dementia?
- Can you assess my home for safety to prevent falls for my loved one with dementia?
- How can I leverage my loved one's remaining capacities?
- How can I enhance my loved one's social participation?

Where to find an occupational therapist?

Occupational therapists work in hospitals, schools, long-term care facilities, rehabilitation centers, mental health facilities, home health care, etc. Ask your family doctor for guidance in finding one.

How to partner with an occupational therapist?

Try the occupational therapist's strategies, even if you initially think they won't work with your loved one. You can only know for sure once you try. Observe the results, document them with observable facts, and report back to the occupational therapist. If another family member lives with you and your loved one with dementia, involve them. Two pairs of eyes are better than one.

PSYCHOLOGIST

Psychologists are mental health professionals specializing in diagnosing and treating emotional, behavioral, and mental health conditions. In dementia care, psychologists play a crucial role in assessing and providing treatment for individuals with dementia while extending support to their caregivers. Psychologists can also perform memory tests to determine whether memory loss is related to dementia or other conditions such as depression.

When and where to find a psychologist?

As soon as you notice early signs of dementia, it's advisable to consult a psychologist. Being a dementia caregiver can be very isolating.

To find a psychologist, use the "APA psychologist locator" (type this keyword in a search engine precisely) and enter your location. Then, in the "Practice areas," you can filter professionals on the "Alzheimer's dementia" criterion. Refrain from overusing filter criteria, though, as this could eliminate potential good fits for your needs. For instance, some psychologists do not label themselves as "Alzheimer's/dementia" specialists, but will list "senior care" among their skills.

When you meet a psychologist for the first time, here are some questions you may want to ask:

- How often should my loved one with dementia consult with you?
- How long is one session?
- Can the sessions take place alternatively online and in person?
- What are realistic expectations for my loved one with dementia and my family?
- Which treatment method best addresses the challenges I face as a caregiver?
- Would joint sessions with my loved one be beneficial?

Medicare might cover family counseling services for your loved one with dementia but not for you as a caregiver. In addition, many psychologists do not accept Medicare or only take private insurance coverage.

How to partner with a psychologist?

Arrive prepared for the initial meeting by describing your loved one's behaviors and emotions, along with your own reactions and coping strategies. Stick to observable facts, avoiding subjective interpretations. Utilize a journal to provide context. Encourage an open exploration of your feelings and thoughts, recognizing their impact on you and your loved one. Remember that emphasizing self-care is crucial while focusing on the therapeutic journey with the psychologist. You may also benefit from exploring available support groups and resources for additional support.

MUSIC THERAPISTS

Music therapists employ music to support individuals with dementia and their caregivers, either individually or together, in addressing challenges related to communication, cognition, motor skills, creativity, emotions, social interaction, and sensory experiences. They craft musical activities to evaluate skills in these seven domains. Using a structured approach, music therapists identify strengths and weaknesses, establish goals, and create a treatment plan. They document session details, observations, and progress toward goals in clinical notes.

Here are some examples of goals and objectives of a music therapist in the cognitive, motor skills, and emotional areas, which are generally prevalent in dementia care:

Cognitive Area:

- Your loved one with dementia: Stimulate memory recall by integrating familiar tunes into daily routines.
- Yourself: Develop personalized playlists to evoke positive memories and initiate discussions.

- Joint Goal: Engage in musical games that enhance cognitive functions, such as identifying song titles or recalling lyrics.

Motor Skills Area:

- Your loved one with dementia: Improve fine motor skills by playing simple instruments.
- Yourself: Encourage a wide range of movements through dance or rhythmic exercises.
- Joint Goal: Enhance coordination by clapping or tapping along with music.

Emotional Area:

- Your loved one with dementia: Allow emotional expression and release through personalized song choices.
- Yourself: Recognize and respond to emotional cues expressed through music.
- Joint Goal: Share emotional experiences through musical storytelling or thematic playlists.

In dementia care, music therapy offers a unique avenue for holistic well-being by contributing to your loved one's (not to mention your own) psychosocial support. Music therapists can play a crucial role within multidisciplinary healthcare teams.

When to consult a music therapist?

Consult a music therapist when you observe signs that music engagement could benefit your loved one with dementia, regardless of the stage or type of dementia. Music therapy offers a unique way to access memories, emotions, and cognitive functions. Music may also foster social connection for you and your loved one with dementia. The goal is to enhance the quality of life and overall well-being for you and your loved one.

What to ask a music therapist?

Key questions to ask a music therapist during your first session:

- Do you have experience with older adults, dementia, and family caregivers?
- Is peer or professional supervision a part of your practice?
- How do you stay updated on evolving theories and clinical practices?
- Do you supervise music therapy interns?

Asking these questions helps ensure you engage with a certified music therapist who is grounded in ethical principles and equipped with evidence-based practices. Accredited music therapists undergo continuous education, which is vital for maintaining their certification.

Where to find a music therapist?

You can connect with a certified music therapist in your area through professional referrals from healthcare providers or self-referrals. You can also visit the Certification Board for Music Therapy (CBMT)'s website at CBMT.org and click "find a therapist."

How to partner with a music therapist?

Starting music therapy sessions can be a meaningful step in your dementia care journey. From the beginning, be open about your intentions, and if you have specific goals in mind, communicate them. If you're unsure, that's perfectly okay — the music therapist is there to collaborate with you, tailoring goals and objectives that benefit your loved one, you, or both of you together.

In cases where your loved one cannot provide informed consent, a humanistic music therapist will diligently craft goals that align with their "probable wishes," respecting their autonomy even in the absence of explicit consent. Beyond addressing your loved one's needs, the therapist will actively support *you* in managing the stress and fatigue that often accompany caregiving, helping you navigate the challenges while maintaining your well-being.

Opting for joint music therapy sessions with your loved one to enhance your relationship has to be rooted in unconditional support. Within this space, both of you are encouraged to express yourselves freely. It's essential to uphold a respectful presence during these sessions, acknowledging the enduring humanity of your loved one. Remember, in this collaborative process, neither the music therapist nor you will treat the sessions as if your loved one is absent. The music therapy environment is intentionally inclusive, meant to foster connection and understanding.

3. CARE COORDINATION AND LEGAL SUPPORT

SOCIAL WORKER

Social workers are the linchpins in your journey, connecting you and your family to doctors, healthcare services, legal and financial aid, and crucial facilities like respite services, senior day programs, assisted living, and skilled nursing facilities. They serve as educators, helping you understand and navigate dementia. They also help you understand your loved one's needs, ensuring they receive the best care and support available.

Social workers also act as mediators, serving as a neutral and impartial point of contact during challenging decisions related to the care of your loved one with dementia. They also assist you in finding support, negotiating with your employer to adapt your job conditions to your caregiver role, and balancing your caregiver duties with other responsibilities. Finally, they also act as family therapists, lending an ear and providing emotional support to alleviate stress.

When to Consult a Social Worker?

As soon as you suspect your loved one may be affected by dementia, consider reaching out to a social worker. These professionals may help you speed up the process of getting a formal dementia diagnosis for your loved one, and then provide support and guidance in nearly every aspect of dementia care. They offer priceless support from the get-go.

What to Ask A Social Worker?

When seeking guidance from a social worker, consider asking these questions:

- What can I expect in regards to my loved one with dementia's behavior in the upcoming weeks and months?

- How can I approach my loved one's employer regarding disability-related benefits and support if they lose their job due to declining performance related to dementia?
- Is it normal that I feel so stressed? What can I do to alleviate stress?
- I need help. Where can I get support or assistance?
- Are there respite services available in my area?
- How can I involve my siblings more in the caregiving process, especially in disagreements?
- How can I join a peer support group for additional assistance and guidance?

These questions aim to provide insights into the progression of your loved one's condition, address personal stress, assist in receiving compensation for the loss of employment due to cognitive decline, identify available support services, navigate family involvement in caregiving, and access additional assistance through support groups. Social workers are equipped to offer guidance and resources in these areas.

Where to Find a Social Worker?

To find a social worker in your area, try looking online for community agencies that offer social work services, mental health clinics, hospitals with specialized dementia care units, nonprofit organizations focusing on elder care. Explore state-funded initiatives, universities, and clinical studies. Also, consider seeking out private social workers or geriatric care managers. Although these options might seem expensive at first glance, in the long run, they may help you save money. Refer to the "Geriatric Care Manager" section in the appendix for more details.

Does Medicare cover Social Work Services?

Medicare usually covers clinical social workers providing counseling, therapy, and outpatient care under Part B. These professionals use their specific qualifications to assist in navigating healthcare systems and complex family dynamics. They also provide mental health support. Often, services like therapy sessions, screenings, and medication management are included. Local resources, like the Area Agency on Aging, can offer additional guidance if you need more information about Medicare coverage.

How to partner with a Social Worker?

Articulate the needs of your loved one at home. Also, share your own challenges: complex family dynamics, exhaustion, financial struggles. Be transparent about your stress level, and seek guidance on stress management techniques. Discuss your daily challenges, and ask the social worker whether or not your objectives and expectations align with your loved one's needs. Remember, effective and open communication is the most important aspect for fruitful collaboration with a social worker.

ELDER LAW ATTORNEY

An elder law attorney specializes in providing legal services for older adults. These attorneys play a significant role in guiding elderly clients through legal and regulatory complexities. Their primary focus is to protect clients' assets, provide for their care, and ensure their wishes are respected as they age.

They address various aspects, including:

- Medicaid Planning, Social Security, and Insurance Claims
- Housing and Long-Term Care
- Wills and Trusts
- Social Security and Retirement
- Elder Abuse
- Inheritance Tax Return Optimization
- Power of Attorney for Dementia (more information below)

Power of attorney

A power of attorney (POA) is a legal document enabling somebody (the principal) to designate a trusted person (the agent), often the primary family caregiver, to make decisions on their behalf when they become incapacitated. This authority typically activates upon receiving the dementia diagnosis.

Power of attorney for healthcare

A healthcare power of attorney allows an individual with dementia to designate a healthcare agent (or proxy) to make medical decisions for them when they become incapacitated to do so themselves. This legal document, also called "medical power of attorney," is an advance directive encompassing critical choices, including selecting doctors, healthcare providers, treatment methods, and care settings.

In the advanced stages of dementia, the healthcare agent may also have to make end-of-life decisions, such as determining whether to provide nutrition through a feeding tube or issuing a do-not-resuscitate (DNR) order to healthcare providers.

Initiating honest and transparent discussions in advance can prevent disagreements and alleviate distress among family members when these decisions need to be made. Anyone of legal age who understands the implications of medical power of attorney can choose an agent, and there is no restriction on who can be appointed.

Conservatorship

Conservatorship, also known as "guardianship" in some states, is a legal relationship in which a court appoints an individual, known as a "conservator" or "guardian," to oversee the personal or financial affairs of an incapacitated person known as a "conservatee" or "ward." The goal of conservatorship is to guarantee that a person's fundamental needs are satisfied, and that their assets are safeguarded when they cannot decide for themselves due to physical or cognitive impairment.

The main distinction between a power of attorney and conservatorship is that the latter is a court-ordered arrangement aiming to protect the rights and assets of an already incapacitated person. In contrast, a power of attorney is a proactive move taken by an individual still capable of making informed decisions to select an agent to act on their behalf.

Living will

Like a healthcare power of attorney, a living will is a type of advance directive. But this time, individuals directly state their preferences for medical care preemptively, before they become incapable of doing so. They don't appoint a healthcare agent to do it on their behalf. A living will includes instructions on employing additional medical procedures and life-sustaining medications, such as artificial nourishment and hydration.

Living will regulations differ from state to state. Thus, speaking with a lawyer familiar with your state's regulations is best. You can see examples of decisions a person with dementia may have to make in a living will at www.dementia-directive.org.

When and where to find an elder law attorney?

Your loved one should see an elder law attorney as early as possible after the dementia diagnosis or even before the diagnosis, when symptoms of dementia, like significant memory loss, start to occur.

To find an elder law attorney, consider using the following resources:

- Your local Alzheimer's Association chapter, or Community Resource Finder.
- The Online directory of the National Academy of Elder Law Attorneys.
- The Eldercare Locator, either online or by calling 1-800-677-1116.
- LawHelp.org for reduced-cost legal aid programs.
- The National Elder Law Foundation. Visit https://nelf.org, scroll over "find a CELA," and click "CELA directory search."

Cost Considerations

Dementia is the most expensive health-related condition in the United States. In its "2023 Alzheimer's Disease Facts and Figures" publication, the Alzheimer's Association stated that the overall lifetime expenses for caring for an individual with dementia amount to almost $400,000; two-thirds of which is borne by caregivers. And, although costs may appear prohibitive for many, hiring an elder law attorney remains advantageous because you can save quite a bit of money elsewhere (tax savings, Medicare/Medicaid claims, etc.). The savings obtained from using an elder law attorney can be proportionately substantial.

To get an idea of the cost of an elder law attorney, it might help to consult the 2022 Forbes Health article entitled, "Hiring an elder law attorney," available online at www.forbes.com/health/healthy-aging/elder-law-attorney.

What to ask an elder law attorney when you meet them for the first time?

- Can you explain the services you typically provide dementia patients and their caregivers?
- Can you provide references or examples of cases you have handled that were similar to mine?
- What is your caseload, and how often are you available?
- Do you collaborate with other professionals to provide comprehensive support to my loved one with dementia, and how?

How to partner with an elder law attorney?

- Make your goals and objectives clear.
- Put effort into finding an excellent elder care attorney. Once you've found the right one, trust them. Do not try to do things your way without professional advice just to save a few hundred dollars, and then come back to them when trouble arises.
- Bring all the appropriate documents, and make sure they are well organized. To help you know which documents to bring, the Alzheimer's Association provides a list at www.alz.org/help-support/caregiving/financial-legal-planning/planning-ahead-for-legal-matters.

4. HOME SUPPORT

ASSISTIVE CARE PERSONNEL

Assistive care personnel are individuals who provide personal care, do some basic housekeeping, and assist your loved one with dementia in their activities of daily living.

They can be Personal Care Aides (PCAs), Home Health Aides (HHAs), or Certified Nurse Assistants (CNAs), with the certified nurse assistant having the highest level of education, and the Personal Care Aide having the lowest.

A PCA is a caregiver who provides non-medical support and assistance to individuals with daily living activities, including bathing, homemaking, shopping, and running errands. A personal care aide does not have formal training or certification.

An HHA is a caregiver who provides personal care services and basic medical care in the patient's home, which may include activities of daily living such as bathing, dressing, toileting, and checking vital signs. A home health aide typically has more training and certification than a personal care aide, and education requirements vary depending on the state. Home health aides may be required to have completed a state-approved training program and passed a competency exam.

A CNA is a healthcare worker who provides basic care to patients in a hospital or nursing home setting. Certified nurse assistants undertake various responsibilities, including monitoring vital signs, personal care, meal service, bed-making, medical equipment setup, observation of patient conditions, infection control, catheter care,and treatment assistance. However, these tasks should be conducted under the supervision of a registered nurse or nurse practitioner. Moreover, becoming a certified nurse assistant necessitates completion of a state-approved training program along with passing a competency exam.

When to hire assistive care personnel?

If, in the course of your dementia caregiving journey, you feel overwhelmed and irritable, it may be time to hire assistive care personnel, or consider finding a day program for your loved one with dementia to attend. You might hesitate to do that because of the cost, the logistics, the discomfort of having someone at your home, or the fear of triggering family conflicts. But in the long run, the benefits outweigh the disadvantages: home care increases the quality of care received, postpones the need for residential care, the house will be more peaceful and safer for everyone, and you'll get the respite time you need to focus on your own health.

What to ask assistive care personnel?

When you're convinced about hiring assistive personnel, prepare your interview questions to verify the person you want to hire is honest and cares for others. Ask them about their training and experience related to dementia care. Finally, make sure their skills are confirmed by someone competent. For instance, seek an RN's supervision to ensure your prospective CNA knows their job.

The first quality of assistive care personnel is to love caring for other people, especially those with special needs. Skills are also necessary, but caring is the most important attribute for this role.

Have a contingency plan when assistive care personnel call in sick or are absent. Ensure this scenario is covered in the contract if you hire personnel through an agency. If you deal with assistive care personnel directly, make sure to have a contract! For more information on contracts, refer to https://www.dementiacarecentral.com/caregiverinfo/personal-care-agreements. Make sure everything is covered in your agreement, including contingency plans. Also, include a formal trial period in your contract, and try to be present during this time so you can observe them.

Where to find assistive care personnel?

To find assistive care personnel:

- Use all the resources listed on this page : https://www.alz.org/help-support/caregiving/care-options/in-home-care
- Do not rush the selection process. This role is critical, so don't take the hiring process lightly. Use all the channels and verifications you can.
- Ask for a referral from your general practitioner.
- Use Medicare's online tool at https://www.medicare.gov/care-compare/?providerType=HomeHealth&redirect=true.
- Use Alzheimer.org community resource finder.
- Find your local Alzheimer's Association chapter, and ask them for different options.
- Search through the eldercare locator at https://eldercare.acl.gov

- Ask your friends and family. Word of mouth from a trustworthy person is often a great place to start. Ensure you have a contract if you hire assistive care personnel through this channel.

Medicare coverage varies a lot when it comes to home care services. Home care services could be covered in full, partly, or not at all, depending on your loved one's coverage. Verify with your loved one with dementia's social worker or a Medicare specialist.

How to partner with an assistive care personnel?

Have a ready-made list of all the needs, and ensure the job conditions are clearly stated. Be respectful and transparent in your expectations. Hope for the best, and prepare for the worst. Also, be honest about your loved one with dementia's behaviors.

At the end of the day, you want the best possible person for them. Assistive care personnel can be a gem or a lemon. In all cases, you want to ensure your loved one with dementia's safety and well-being, while at the same time, cover your own back.

DAY CENTERS

Day centers, sometimes called "adult daycares," provide your loved one with dementia the opportunity to participate in supervised social activities so you can have some time for self care. The goals of a day center are generally to break up isolation through activities and socialization, to maintain the autonomy of seniors, and to support their caregivers. The team caring for your loved one in a day center may include physical, occupational, speech, and creative arts (music, art, dance-movement, drama) therapists, special educators, rehabilitation assistants or orderlies, and registered nurses.

Adult daycares are one of the most essential resources to support families. They offer services to individuals with dementia, even in the moderate stage. But they generally don't tolerate behaviors that can jeopardize the cohesion and safety of a group, such as aggressive behaviors, for instance. If a person requires frequent one-on-one assistance, their application might be rejected.

Day centers generally provide healthy meals and transportation from home to the day center and back. Staff is trained to provide physical and psychosocial support, stimulate your loved one with dementia cognitively and physically, and facilitate social interactions with peers.

When and where to apply for participation in a day center?

Applying to a day center is best in early dementia, as your loved one will get used to the place and staff before symptoms worsen. The sooner, the better. To find a day center that's right for your loved one with dementia, consider using the resources below:

- The Alzheimer's Association dedicates a whole section to day centers at https://www.alz.org/help-support/caregiving/care-options/adult-day-centers.
- The community resource finder at https://www.communityresourcefinder.org/. Click on "COMMUNITY SERVICES", select "Adult Day Care Programs" among the list of services, then specify your area.
- https://www.nadsa.org/locator/

Note: Some day centers may assess their prospective participants directly at home. Before registering your loved one in a day center, you might want to ask the following questions to the management:

- Does the staff have dementia care training or experience?
- Does the day center have a weekly program of activities? Can I choose activities for my loved one based on their immediate interests and needs?
- What are the hours of attendance?
- How much does the program cost?

Though original Medicare generally does not cover the cost of a day center, Medicaid does in some states. Government programs for veterans may also cover the cost of a day center.

How to partner with the day center staff?

- Be honest about your loved one with dementia's desire to attend the day center and their level of independence.
- Provide your loved one's family history.
- Provide staff with relevant tips and strategies for your loved one with dementia.
- Collaborate to the best of your ability to facilitate your loved one with dementia's integration.
- Be available to answer the staff's questions.
- You might want to provide a small reminder (or, for spouses, a love letter) so the staff can read it to reassure your loved one with dementia. This strategy may calm anxiety if they try to "go back home" or look for you.

To conclude this chapter, remember that all these professionals won't be involved simultaneously. Their intervention is guided by the functional needs and level of independence your loved one with dementia still has. Thus, one rule of thumb is to carefully observe and methodically document the evolution of your loved one's symptoms and behaviors. Doing this will help you and your dream team of professionals determine the approaches and actions that will best serve your loved one's interests. In addition, this will make you feel useful to your loved one's helpers – organized, attentive, caring, and resilient – which is precisely the kind of caregiver you are, given you are reading this book!

CHAPTER 6

JOINING FORCES WITH FAMILY AND FRIENDS

"Anything is possible when you have the right people there to support you."

— Misty Copeland

Jennifer has always been very close to her mother, and had no problem accepting the responsibility to care for her. However, since Lovely was diagnosed with dementia, Jennifer has had to make significant sacrifices, including balancing work and family life with her role as a caregiver to ensure Lovely receives the care and support she needs.

Despite the challenges and stresses of caring for someone with dementia, Jennifer is deeply devoted to her mother and determined to make her daily life as comfortable and fulfilling as possible. She works tirelessly to keep her mother engaged and active.

John too, like his sister Jennifer, has always been close to his mother. He loved helping his mom on her farm, and exploring the vast fields and forests surrounding their home. He would often spend hours wandering through the lush greenery, marveling at the beauty of nature and the countless wonders it held.

As he grew up, despite his mother's love and support, John was not content with their humble life, and longed for something more. He dreamed of metropolitan life, of finding an excellent job in the city, and being able to provide for his mother in a way she had never known. Finally, he gathered the courage to leave home in pursuit of his dream.

Years later, John had become the city guy he imagined. He sat at his desk, staring blankly at his computer screen, but couldn't focus on the project before him. His mind was constantly drifting back to his mother, who had been diagnosed with dementia a few years ago. Since that time, it has been a difficult journey for their family. He loved his mother deeply, but his job as a high-powered executive took up most of his time and energy. He couldn't remember the last time he had visited his mom at Jennifer's home where she now lived.

John's heart ached with guilt as he thought about how much he missed her. The thought of his mom's sharp mind slowly declining, and the possibility that she might not remember him one day, was too much to bear. He made a mental note to schedule a visit as soon as possible.

But as the days passed, John got caught up in work again. Meetings, conference calls, and deadlines consumed his every thought. He meant to visit his mother and sister; he truly did, but time seemed to slip away from him.

One day, John received a call from Jennifer. His sister explained that she was worried about the recent changes with their mom, so she started having a nurse visit them at home. John felt a rush of panic and fear. He couldn't bear it any longer. He quickly gathered his things and left for home. The office would have to wait.

John packed some things for an extended visit to see his mom. On the drive down to his sister's house, he couldn't shake the feeling of regret, and wished he had been there for her more. He knew he couldn't change the past, but vowed to make it up to her in the present.

Like Jennifer and John, you may have unequal support from certain family members or friends. You may have issues with communication, or worse yet, the relationship with them might deteriorate because of disagreements. On the contrary, they may be willing to help, but are incapable of acting efficiently due to grief and sadness. In that case, they may just need guidance. And that's why we included this chapter. To help you look at ways to join forces with family and friends when you have a loved one with dementia.

ANNOUNCING THE DIAGNOSIS TO FAMILY MEMBERS AND FRIENDS

It is not uncommon to see family caregivers delay announcing a dementia diagnosis to other close family members. Caregivers are sometimes ashamed or afraid of how their siblings will react. Sometimes, family members become confused, upset, deeply saddened, or skeptical. Still, others may be sympathetic, and offer help right from the beginning.

Upon receiving a dementia diagnosis, families often rally together, offering support that brings comfort to the affected person, resolving old conflicts, and fostering a sense of unity. However, as dementia advances, new tensions might arise, altering family dynamics significantly. The evolving caregiving roles and increasing demands can be daunting. Yet, with careful planning and preparation, families can navigate these challenges, emerging stronger than ever, transcending the impact of the diagnosis. Although it may be difficult for other family members to fully grasp the impact dementia has on your loved one (and you, as their primary caregiver), good communication can aid their understanding.

Inform your family about your loved one's condition and current dementia stage, explaining the implications. Communicate any changes you notice in their condition. Involve family members when you need additional support or specific tasks to be completed. Share discoveries that improve your loved one's well-being with them. Stress the value of teamwork and effective communication in enhancing caregiving efforts. Invite them to a dementia support group session. Hearing other caregivers talk about their daily challenges can be a real eye-opener, and a helpful reality check.

UNITING FAMILY MEMBERS IN DEMENTIA CAREGIVING

Navigating the caregiving journey is a path best traveled together as a united family. Somebody in the family has to take the leadership role in gathering siblings together for an open and heartfelt conversation. In this safe space, thoughts and concerns can be freely shared.

Here is some advice on how to lead that conversation:

- **Recognize each sibling's unique strengths**, availability, and circumstances, appreciating the diverse contributions they can make.
- **Build a plan**, write it down, and define roles and responsibilities.
- Consider the **financial and legal aspects**, ensuring decisions are collectively made.
- **Assign caregiving tasks**, from medical appointments to emotional support, tailoring responsibilities to fit each sibling's capabilities and commitments (refer to Chapter 4).
- Design a **shared calendar** or schedule to harmonize visits and caregiving duties, promoting collaboration and understanding.
- Regular communication is the cornerstone—establish a **channel for updates and discussions**, fostering adaptability as your loved one's condition evolves.
- **Periodically review and adjust** your caregiving plan, and above all, advocate for self-care.
- Encourage each sibling to **prioritize their own well-being**; a well-nurtured caregiver provides the best care (refer to Chapter 2).

It is possible for gratitude to flow freely among siblings for the efforts and love they invest: "Thank you for being there," "Thank you for being you," "I appreciate all the love and care you've been providing," "I'm grateful to have you in my life," " Your kindness has brightened my day," "You touched my heart" can all make a big difference.

WHAT TO DO WHEN THE FAMILY DOES NOT AGREE ON THE CARE TO GIVE?

Such scenarios are pervasive; they happen in every family. Encourage each person to express their concerns and perspectives openly while emphasizing the best interests of your loved one. Understanding and empathizing with varying viewpoints is crucial. Aim for compromises that accommodate different preferences and capabilities. Try to bring facts instead of emotions. Sit down, write out the problems, and find a way to get rid of negative feelings. Make it clear that it's a sacrifice everybody has to make. And that everyone needs to put aside their ego and dreams of a perfect situation that does not exist. You must find the positive sides everyone has to bring, and verbally let them know that you noticed. Hearing these positive and constructive statements can benefit your loved one with dementia.

Involving the person with dementia in decision-making, if possible, and documenting agreed-upon care plans help maintain clarity and unity. Additionally, educating family members about dementia and caregiving approaches fosters informed decision-making, while acknowledging and respecting individual limits and contributions is essential for effective collaboration. Ultimately, keeping the focus on providing the best care for your loved one unites the family in a common goal. Seeking the assistance of a professional mediator or counselor can provide neutral guidance and facilitate consensus, if necessary.

But of course, if your family does not help, support groups are a great option to share your challenges and find solutions from other people's experiences. Participating in support groups, seeking guidance from a counselor or pastor, or exploring care possibilities can provide valuable assistance throughout your journey. Remember, you're not facing this alone.

WHAT TO DO WHEN OLD FAMILY STORIES COME BACK TO DAMAGE RELATIONSHIPS?

It can be hard to let go of the past. People's ideas and decisions can be significantly impacted by challenging events, among other aspects of their daily lives. And it's no different when you have old histories with a loved one with dementia.

However, there are ways to address the lingering effects of past experiences. Practicing self-compassion, having a neutral space for discussion, utilizing mindfulness to focus on the present moment, finding an intermediary, or seeking therapy are possible ways to manage these unresolved feelings. And, just as a side-note, in situations where words aren't enough or the burden is too heavy, music can be an invaluable tool to use. As I saw in my practice, songwriting can help you express what you experience as you support your loved one with dementia.

SANDWICH CAREGIVER: HOW TO FIND BALANCE

Being a "sandwich" caregiver, or "sandwich generation" caregiver means caring for your kids and your loved one with dementia simultaneously, with everyone living in the same house. In this position, you may struggle with caring for your loved one with dementia, children at home, career, self-care, and household tasks.

Several approaches may help you address these concerns and reduce the stress and pressure associated with multiple responsibilities.

Recognize the Most Urgent Need

As a dementia caregiver, you're often managing multiple tasks - aiding your teenager with a homework assignment, feeding the dog, and attending to Mom's restlessness. It becomes essential to prioritize urgent and important matters first. Focus on addressing that singular task, devising alternate strategies for handling the remaining obligations (perhaps you help your teenager with his assignment first, then come to mom's aid while asking your teenager to feed the dog).

I like to use the Eisenhower matrix (named after the former president) to organize my duties. Perhaps it could also help you prioritize your tasks.

Eisenhower matrix

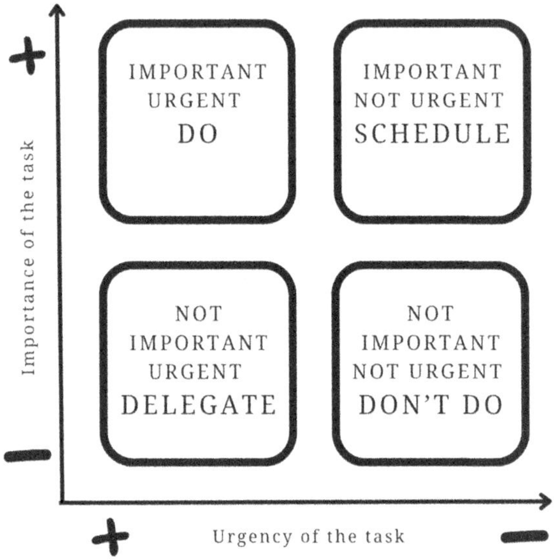

The vertical axis indicates the importance of the task, and the horizontal axis indicates its time-sensitiveness; the further up, the more critical, and the further left, the more urgent. In the top-left area, put all the essential tasks you must complete as soon as possible. The vital duties to spread over time with deadlines will go in the top-right corner. In the bottom left, arrange the tasks you can do later in the day when things slow down a bit. And, in the bottom-right, list things you'd like to do, whenever you get around to it. Finally, ask yourself if you even have to complete the bottom-right tasks. If so, do them in your free time; if not, do yourself a favor, and eliminate them.

Enlist All Family Members in Helping with Care

Unfortunately, many caregivers are disappointed that family members aren't interested in taking on their fair share of caregiving responsibilities. Notwithstanding, members of the family including children, can learn precious life lessons by helping provide age-appropriate levels of care for your loved one, most of the time their grandmother or grandfather. For instance, simple tasks such as reading a book together or drawing with their grandparents create opportunities for bonding and allow you some moments to recharge.

Ask for and Accept Help

Be specific when you ask for help, to avoid the generic: "If you need anything, let me know." People generally mean well, but very often need guidance on what to do. Once friends and other family members know the stress you're facing by caring for your loved one with dementia (children at home, career, self-care, and household tasks), they usually want to help out, but are unsure how.

When someone offers assistance, respond appreciatively with a "Yes, thank you!" and suggest various tasks you could use help with, such as laundry, grocery shopping, slicing and portioning vegetables, walking the dog, or even spending time with your loved one. If no one extends a helping hand, consider approaching those nearest to you, openly acknowledging your need for support, and being clear about the kind of assistance you require.

INGREDIENTS FOR HARMONIOUS FAMILY RELATIONSHIPS AND FRIENDSHIPS

Improving the recipe for harmonious relationships takes a lifetime, but some key ingredients are needed. Love is the root of all positive interactions. If there is love, though not perfect love, you may implement the following concrete actions to create harmony:

- **Open, honest, and respectful communication** is the foundation of any healthy relationship. It involves active listening (rephrasing what you heard to be sure you understood), expressing oneself clearly, and being receptive to one another's thoughts and feelings.
- **Speak kindly to each other**. This may seem obvious, but when we are under pressure or busy, we frequently say things we don't mean, or adopt a tone that offends others. Apologize if your words or tone hurt someone you love. Explain that your behavior was unintended, and that you are under pressure; which has nothing to do with them. Tell them you will do your best to speak more gently in the future.
- **Value the uniqueness of each member of your family**. You value family uniqueness more than you think. Identify your family members' characteristics that you find interesting, unique, or even wonderful, and celebrate them. Doing this strengthens your family bonds.
- **Spend quality time** together. Whether through shared activities, meals, or meaningful conversations, dedicating time to nurture relationships creates lasting memories and deepens family ties.
- **Cultivating empathy** allows individuals to put themselves in another's shoes, understand their perspective, and respond compassionately. Understanding each other's emotions and experiences fosters stronger bonds.
- **Trust** is the foundation of any meaningful relationship. Reliability, keeping promises, and demonstrating integrity build trust and strengthen the connection between individuals.
- **Forgiveness** is the key to any relationship. Letting go of misunderstandings or conflicts and having the resilience to bounce back from challenges helps maintain a positive and lasting connection. Forgiveness showcases a higher level of maturity in the human journey.

When practiced and nurtured, these ingredients contribute to harmonious and fulfilling family relationships and friendships.

FRIENDSHIPS IN DIFFICULT DAYS ARE SO PRECIOUS

Friendship is crucial in our lives, and while some people find it easier to make and keep friends than others, we all need good friends to surround us. Some personal characteristics are essential for cultivating healthy, lasting friendships, especially in challenging times. Here are a few traits that can influence relationships:

- **Trustworthiness** is the "make or break" factor in every interpersonal interaction. Any break in trust can destroy a connection, no matter how minor. Have honest conversations, apologize for past mistakes, and practice patience in your relationships.
- **Dependability**: Being dependable means your friends can rely on you to keep and carry out your promises. Sometimes, your busy schedule related to your loved one with dementia might cause you to miss meetings with your friends. Keep communication open with them so they understand what's going on.
- **Loyalty**: From the moment we form our first connections, loyalty is essential in all relationships. We need friends who won't reveal our personal information to others, spread rumors about us, or let others judge us. And the same goes for us. Surround yourself only with loyal friends, and act the same way for them. You have enough on your plate already with caring for your loved one with dementia to risk entering into conflicts with good friends.
- **Humor** is exceptionally precious for building and maintaining relationships. It helps reduce stress, create a positive environment, and improve communication. The only word of caution is to use it respectfully and appropriately. The last thing you want is to hurt your friends' feelings at a time when you need their support.

- **Self-mockery** refers to using humor and irony to get through the trials and difficulties of caring for a person with dementia. Some examples of self-deprecation include joking about forgetfulness, confusion, or other symptoms of dementia and poking fun at one's own struggles and frustrations as a caregiver. Self-deprecation can be a powerful coping mechanism in support groups because peers can understand exactly where it comes from. Remember, while self-mockery can be a healthy way to cope with the stresses of dementia care, ensure that it does not become hurtful or disrespectful towards your loved one with dementia.

CARING FOR A DEMENTIA PARENT, EVEN IF THEY WEREN'T A GOOD PARENT TO YOU AS A CHILD

Caring for a loved one with dementia is even more challenging if your loved one with dementia did not treat you kindly in the past. Remember that dementia can change a person's behavior, and they may be unable to recall their actions. Therefore, try your best to approach the situation with a clean slate, extending empathy and understanding. Recognize and accept your feelings of resentment, hurt, or anger from your past experiences. It's crucial to acknowledge these emotions as a valid part of your journey.

Secondly, remember your "WHY," and own it. Why did you choose to care for your loved one with dementia in the first place? You could have just dropped them at the entrance to the hospital or long-term care facility and let the system take care of them. But you didn't. Thus, honestly ask yourself, why?

There are many reasons to care for someone other than reciprocating what they did for us. Maybe you want to show an example of solidarity to your children, to your community, to respect your oath at your wedding (sickness and health), or follow what the Bible says, "respect your parents," etc. You can always find a reason higher than your past challenges and pain; but establish clear boundaries to protect your own well-being. Determine what you can and cannot handle regarding caregiving responsibilities and emotional engagement. Finally, consider consulting a therapist or counselor to help you process and deal with your emotions. They can provide guidance and coping mechanisms tailored to your situation.

GRIEVING: A FAMILY TRIAL

Grieving as a family is a challenging and emotional journey. Still, there are ways to support each other through the process.

Here are some pieces of advice to navigate the grieving process together:

- Understand that **everyone grieves differently**. Some may want to discuss their feelings, while others need space and time alone.
- Recognize that **grief takes time**, and family members may process their emotions differently. Exercise patience and understanding, allowing each person to heal at their own pace.
- **Be kind to yourself and your siblings**. Small gestures of kindness and compassion can go a long way in providing emotional support.
- If the grief becomes overwhelming or prolonged, consider seeking the help of a **grief counselor or therapist**. Professional support can provide coping strategies and facilitate the healing process.
- Establish family rituals or **create memorials** to honor and remember your loved one. Keep the memory of the loved one alive through prayers, traditions, dedications, or acts of generosity in their name. Create a legacy that carries on their values and spirit.
- Take **one day at a time**, emphasizing the importance of rest, proper nutrition, exercise, and engaging in activities that bring joy and relaxation.
- Consider joining a **grief support group** as a family, or a support group for others currently caring for a loved one

with dementia. Sharing experiences with others who have gone through similar paths or losses can be comforting and provide additional perspectives.

Supporting each other through grief is an ongoing process. Encourage empathy, love, and understanding within the family to help each member heal and find comfort during this difficult phase. In times of loss, emotions can be overwhelming, especially when roles shift after a loved one with dementia passes away. If a sibling becomes the will's executor, even though you've been the primary caregiver, it's natural to feel pushed out and resentful, which can be even more painful. Emotions may run high, but try expressing negative feelings outside family gatherings to avoid unnecessary drama.

Remember, life continues with those who are still here, so resist the urge to isolate yourself. Grieving can be challenging, causing divisions in feelings, but it can also bring brothers, sisters, and parents together. We can acknowledge mistakes, forgive, and renew love by honoring memories. It's a precious opportunity to move forward with a lighter heart.

In this chapter, we saw how revealing the diagnosis to siblings and friends can trigger a range of emotions, from fear and embarrassment, to curiosity and support. As the journey advances and familial roles shift, conflicts may surface, testing the resilience of family bonds. Effective communication, empathy, and an emphasis on facts over emotions can aid in navigating these challenges. Addressing past family wounds and nurturing friendships are pivotal pillars of understanding and maturity. During the grieving phase following the loss of a loved one with dementia, approaching the whirlwind of emotions with compassion and openly accepting/expressing feelings can facilitate healing, allowing the family to embrace the future with a lighter spirit.

CHAPTER 7
PRECIOUS PEERS AND SUPPORT GROUPS

"The simple act of caring is heroic."
— Edward Albert

Despite her brother being as supportive as possible, calling at frequent intervals, sending money intermittently, and helping her to hire a care nurse, Jennifer still had more than she felt like she could handle in the care of her mother. She had been feeling so overwhelmed and isolated with the constant demands of caregiving, compounded with family responsibilities, that things were starting to take an emotional toll on her. Lovely's condition had already progressed to a point where she required round-the-clock care, and Jennifer struggled to balance her responsibilities as a caregiver with her job, her family, and her own needs.

She had heard that there were support groups for dementia caregivers, but figured it would be pointless to join one. Jennifer felt embarrassed and ashamed about her mother's condition, and didn't want to share her personal experiences with strangers. She already felt alone with her family in the struggle, and couldn't relate to anyone else anyway. She didn't have time to attend meetings, and didn't see how adding one more thing to her busy schedule could possibly help.

But Jennifer's condition worsened as time passed, and she began to feel more isolated. She was exhausted, both physically and emotionally. Her marriage was suffering, her relationship with her children was also affected, and she was struggling to cope with the constant demands of her mother's care.

One day, while at a doctor's appointment for her mom, the physician suggested that Jennifer look into support groups for dementia caregivers. At first, she was hesitant, but the doctor assured her that it could benefit her *and* her mother. So she decided to try it out.

She found a support group that met once a week at a local community center, and at her first meeting, Jennifer was surprised to see how many group members had similar experiences. They shared their struggles, successes, and tips on how to deal with the challenges of caregiving. Jennifer was touched when one of the members told her she was not alone, and there were others who truly understood what she was going through.

By participating in the support group, Jennifer learned how to take better care of herself, and developed a sense of control over her situation. She felt less isolated and more connected to others who were going through the same challenges. The support group provided her with a space to talk about her mother's condition and the emotional burden it was placing on her. She found comfort in knowing that she wasn't alone in her struggles and that others were there to walk alongside her.

Participation in the support group was a turning point for Jennifer. She felt more positive and better equipped to face the challenges of caregiving for her mother. She was able to find a balance between her caregiving responsibilities and her own needs. She also noticed that her relationships with her husband and children were improving, as she was becoming more patient and less stressed.

Jennifer realized that joining the support group was one of the best decisions she had ever made. It provided her with valuable support from other caregivers, helping her navigate the challenges of caregiving. She realized that it was not a solitary journey, and that the additional help and support were invaluable tools. Now, Jennifer frequently advocates for caregivers to consider joining a support group, emphasizing the essential role it can play in transforming their caregiving experience. In this chapter, we will look into support groups, their purpose, and the benefits of joining one.

WHAT ARE DEMENTIA CAREGIVER SUPPORT GROUPS?

Dementia caregiver support groups are gatherings where individuals facing similar life challenges, namely caring for a loved one with dementia, come together for mutual understanding and support. These groups provide a safe and sympathetic environment for participants to discuss their struggles, share experiences, and offer advice and encouragement to one another.

They are sometimes led by professionals but, more often, by other dementia caregivers who guide the discussion and ensure everyone has a chance to participate. Hearing about the experiences of others can help individuals feel less alone in their struggles and give them hope in overcoming their challenges.

HOW OFTEN DO SUPPORT GROUPS MEET?

Support groups can meet at different frequencies depending on the organization. Some support groups meet weekly, while others may gather every day of the week, or once a month. In some cases, support groups may have a set schedule. In others, the schedule may be more flexible and determined by the group members. How frequently support groups meet can vary depending on the group's focus and the members' needs. Search different support groups and find one that meets on a schedule that works for you.

ONLINE OR IN-PERSON SUPPORT GROUPS?

Caregivers have various options for support groups. Online groups provide convenience and anonymity by allowing participation from home at any time. In-person groups offer a more personal experience, and foster face-to-face connections. Choose based on your preferences and circumstances. Here's a quick overview of the advantages and disadvantages of both:

ONLINE SUPPORT GROUPS	
PROS	**CONS**
• Easy 24/7 access • Quick information retrieval • Variety of responses to specific questions • Global connections	• Less personal atmosphere • Limited spontaneous sharing • Less impact on stress and burden perception
FACE-TO-FACE SUPPORT GROUPS	
PROS	**CONS**
• Human warmth improves mental and spiritual health • A stronger sense of belonging • More frequent and deeper informal conversations • Physical interactions and demonstrations • Socialization • Research indicates a more significant impact on depression, health, and well-being	• Time-consuming travel • Potential guilt for not attending • Social pressure may keep you in meetings, even when you feel you are not gaining anything from them • Availability may vary based on location

WHERE TO FIND ONLINE SUPPORT GROUPS?

Various online support groups cover a range of topics. You can find them with ease by using:

- Google Search: Type "dementia support groups online" for free options. Results may include dedicated pages or refer you to social media platforms.
- Alzheimer's Online Communities: Explore alzheimer.org's event search tool at https://www.alz.org/events/event_search?etid=2&cid=0.
- Social Media Platforms: Check Facebook, Instagram, TikTok, and similar platforms for relevant support groups.

Where to Find Face-to-Face Support Groups?

Discover in-person dementia support groups through these channels:

- Alzheimer's Association website: Use their event search tool to locate groups facilitated by trained leaders.
- Local Alzheimer's Association chapters: Check for support groups that meet in your area.
- Daycare centers and assisted living facilities: These may host support groups for dementia caregivers.
- Hospitals and clinics: Look for support groups for individuals with dementia and their family members.
- Senior and community centers: Find support groups catering to older adults and caregivers.
- Parkinson's Foundation: Explore their support groups available in many areas.
- Veteran Affairs caregiver support groups: If you or your loved one are veterans, contact the National Caregiver Support Line established by the U.S. Department of Veterans Affairs for assistance.
- Mental Health America: Discover peer-led or professionally-led support groups.

Organize your schedule to attend regularly, and consider seeking assistance for your loved one during the meetings for your own peace of mind.

DEMENTIA SUPPORT GROUPS: EXPLORING COMMON HESITATIONS CAREGIVERS MAY HAVE

Joining a support group might not be an immediate choice for many caregivers. Let's explore some common reasons why you, as a caregiver, may feel hesitant.

- **Juggling time**: With the ever-increasing demands that you face as a caregiver with additional job pressures, carving out a fraction of your hectic schedule to make time for a support group could be difficult. Looking at your job, daily activities with your loved one with dementia, and general responsibilities (children, etc.), you may think a support group won't be a good fit for you.
- **Feeling exhausted or overwhelmed**: With all your responsibilities as a caregiver, you might worry that adding a support group to your schedule could be overwhelming. You may feel that fatigue might make it challenging to engage in certain activities or take on additional commitments.
- **Doubting the benefits of support groups**: It is common for caregivers to question the value of support groups. If you are well-supported by family or a trusted psychotherapist, you may feel you don't need "another group." If deeply rooted in your faith or spirituality, you might worry that discussing stressors could intensify their impact on your life.

To shed light on this, consider the wisdom shared in the Bible. Proverbs 18:21 warns about the power of words, and emphasizes their impact on our lives. The apostle Paul, in Philippians 4:8, encourages focusing on positive thoughts.

Another perspective comes from the Cherokee legend of the two wolves within, illustrating that the one you "feed" more will prevail. From one support group to another, some individuals might confuse "sharing their problems" with "dwelling on them." Venting your feelings is a healthy way to seek support, while dwelling on them could result in a perpetual cycle of negativity without actively working toward a solution.

- **Avoiding others' experiences**: You might be afraid to listen to the stories and experiences out of anxiety that those things may also happen to you or your loved one with dementia.
- **Battling embarrassment or shame**: Despite most support groups being safe spaces, the stigma often attached to dementia may make you uncomfortable sharing about your loved one. Feelings of guilt or shame may stop you from speaking about your experience.
- **Questioning trust**: As a caregiver, you may encounter situations where trust is challenging, even when no specific reason for doubt exists. It's a common human experience, and these doubts can extend to healthcare professionals and other caregivers who participate in support groups.
- **Fearing evaluation:** You might be afraid of being judged on your story or feel uncomfortable speaking about your difficulties. You may be anxious about meeting new people, or talking to strangers about personal issues.
- **Avoiding social groups**: You may never have liked groups as an individual; you feel better alone, and don't have the urge to leave your house often or to be around other people in general.
- **Seeking information:** As a caregiver, you may need help finding and inquiring about the available support groups in your area. If manipulating technology and browsing the Internet is easier said than done for you, finding a convenient support group for your needs may be even more challenging.
- **Favoring individualized support:** You may prefer the option of one-on-one support from a therapist or counselor rather than joining a group.

JOINING DEMENTIA SUPPORT GROUPS WITH CONFIDENCE

Your concerns about joining a dementia support group are valid. The following section doesn't aim to dismiss those concerns or force reasons why support groups are magical solutions for dementia caregivers. Instead, it is meant to provide a different perspective, empowering you to approach support groups with confidence and an open mind.

- **Saving time down the line**: Allocating a portion of your hectic schedule to a support group can be a long-term time-saving strategy. Consider the wealth of combined knowledge and experience related to dementia within the group. Exposure to scientific expertise and practical insights from professional healthcare providers and fellow caregivers can result in more efficient and informed decision-making, providing a valuable return on your invested time.
- **Recharging and boosting your wellness**: Engaging in a support group is a form of self-care. Scientific studies indicate that assisting others, even amid personal challenges, stimulates brain regions linked to pleasure, social connection, and trust. In undertaking the noble endeavor of building a community of mutual support, you not only alleviate the weight of dementia caregiving collectively, but also enhance your overall well-being.
- **Connecting dementia caregivers beyond doubt**: Seeking support from family or a trusted therapist is helpful. Still, support groups offer a unique understanding of your dementia caregiving journey. It may be the only place where you feel fully understood.

If discussing challenges induces guilt or fear due to your faith, consider faith-based support groups. Some incorporate prayers, aligning support with your beliefs. These groups echo the wisdom of the Bible: Matthew 18:20 highlights the power of collective strength, and Galatians 6:2 encourages sharing burdens. A supportive group characterized by kindness, empathy, and unwavering care can transform shared struggles into hope, thus feeding the righteous wolf from the aforementioned Cherokee legend. Joining a support group isn't just about sharing challenges, but about finding understanding and strength in unity on your caregiving journey.

- **Finding comfort in shared journeys**: It's natural to worry about what you might hear in a support group, especially when dealing with the challenges of dementia caregiving. But remember, each journey is unique, and others' experiences don't predict your own. On the contrary, hearing others' stories might offer a fresh perspective, showing your situation isn't as desperate as you thought. Life will continue, and you may gain new insights. Support groups provide differing perspectives, empathy, and practical coping strategies. Take your time to find one that feels right for you.
- **Embracing support without embarrassment or shame**: Joining a support group might feel daunting due to the stigma around dementia, but remember, these groups are safe spaces with minimal judgment. Other group members understand your struggles. It's not about shame, but mutual support. Consider support groups as a sanctuary where your journey is respected and your story helps break down the dementia stigma. Your experience is valuable and contributes to building a compassionate community.
- **Navigating trust**: Building trust is a gradual process, especially if past experiences have left you wary. In a support group, many share similar feelings, fostering understanding and empathy. You're not alone in these concerns. Consider taking small steps, like attending a few sessions to observe before actively participating. Trust evolves through shared stories and genuine support. It's okay to express your concerns within the group—shared vulnerability often builds trust. Each caregiver's journey is

unique, and trust is a personal journey, not a one-size-fits-all solution.

- **Overcoming the fear of being evaluated**: Concerns or discomfort about being judged are valid reactions you might have. The fear of exposing yourself to total strangers is natural. But remember that within the group, caregivers share similar experiences and challenges. Rather than judgment, you'll likely encounter empathy and like-mindedness. Here again, take your time. Sit in a few sessions just to observe before actively participating. The shared vulnerability within the group often leads to an atmosphere of connection and support.
- **Receiving support beyond social norms**: Choosing solitude over social groups is valid, especially in dementia caregiving. Yet, support groups offer more than typical social interactions. They break isolation, creating a community where others truly understand your experiences. They provide practical help, mutual support, and a judgment-free space. They also allow you to invest in your own well-being and find a community that respects your unique journey. Joining a support group is not about becoming social, but about uncovering a supportive community tailored to your specific challenges.
- **Finding information**: Navigating the vast landscape of support groups through online search engines may seem like a formidable task, especially if you are not particularly tech-savvy. However, there are resources available to guide you. Local community centers, healthcare providers, or even a quick call to a dementia helpline or your Alzheimer's Association local chapter can provide information on suitable support groups. Feel free to ask for help or clarification; these resources are here to assist you in finding proper support tailored to your needs. Stay positive. With time and perseverance, you will find a support group that meets your criteria.

COMBINING SUPPORT APPROACHES FOR AN ENRICHED CAREGIVER JOURNEY

Preferring one-on-one support is understandable, but attending a support group doesn't mean giving up individual counseling. Both can harmonize to enrich your caregiving experience. Support groups offer a unique community, shared experiences, and a sense of belonging. Individual counseling provides personalized guidance and tailored strategies. Combining both creates a robust support network, comprehensively addressing different aspects of your caregiving journey.

In the intricate landscape of dementia caregiving, embracing support groups emerges as a strategic anchor. Although joining a support group may raise understandable concerns about time management, exhaustion, and trust, the profound benefits of these groups are undeniable. These communities serve as reservoirs of collective wisdom, offering practical insights that can streamline decision-making over time.

More than just a pragmatic solution, engaging in these groups is a fundamental act of self-care, rewarding its members with enhanced positivity, social connection, and trust. Support groups also provide a unique and nuanced understanding of your caregiving journey, thus supplementing other forms of support. Embracing support groups is an investment in streamlined caregiving and personal well-being by providing a community uniquely attuned to your journey.

CHAPTER 8
WHAT ABOUT YOUR JOB

"Being deeply loved by someone gives you strength while loving someone deeply gives you courage."
—Lao Tzu

Jennifer has constantly been searching for ways to reduce her mother's suffering, while getting the best out of her time.

She continued to care for her mom in every possible way, but at the same time struggled to balance her own responsibilities with her family and her job.

Jennifer works full-time and manages a team. She has been doing her best to keep up with her work by trying to include family members in the care, hiring a visiting nurse, and joining a support group. Yet, she still finds it hard to focus. She constantly worries about her mother and feels guilty for being unable to always be with her.

Jennifer's boss noticed that her work performance had been slipping recently, and that she'd been absent from work more than usual. Her boss suggested taking a break or hiring a caregiver for her mother.

Still, Jennifer was hesitant to leave her mother alone with a stranger all day. She felt her mother needed her, and didn't want to let her down.

Jennifer had been struggling with whether or not to keep leaving her mother at home to go to work when the care nurse wasn't there yet. She felt guilty for wanting to return to her everyday life, and that she was failing as a daughter and as a caregiver. She felt torn between her responsibilities as a working professional and taking care of her mom.

After much deliberation, Jennifer decided to speak to her boss again, but this time, she had a plan. She proposed working flexible hours, starting earlier and finishing later so she could care for her mother during the day. She also suggested working from home to be available for her mother when needed.

Jennifer's boss was impressed by her dedication and willingness to find a solution. He agreed to her proposal, and Jennifer felt a weight lifted off her shoulders. She still felt torn between her job and her responsibilities as a caregiver, but was confident she had found a way to balance both.

Jennifer's story is a reminder that simultaneously being a caregiver and professional can be a challenging and stressful experience. Still, it's essential to communicate with your employer and find a solution that works for everyone.

Balancing your responsibilities as a caregiver and your job is possible with some knowledge and flexibility.

YOUR JOB: A KEY REVENUE STREAM AND SOCIAL LINK

Your job can play a significant role in both generating funds and creating social connections for you as a caregiver.

As a critical revenue stream, your employment can provide you with a steady income, which you can use to support yourself, your family, and your loved one with dementia.

Being a family caregiver entails financial and non-financial burdens. The non-financial consequences include adverse effects on the caregiver's physical, emotional, and social welfare. On the other hand, the economic costs involve various aspects:

- **Employment**: Nearly seven in ten of family caregivers strive to manage the requirements of their job alongside caregiving duties. 25% caregivers has faced considerable alterations in their work circumstances, affecting their earnings. These changes may encompass reduced working hours, taking time off work, job loss, or even early retirement. Moreover, they might also grapple with the loss of their loved one's income due to their illness or disability.
- As a family caregiver, you have the responsibility of **purchasing items** that can aid your loved one with dementia in maintaining their independence. These may include mobility assistance devices, supplies for managing urinary incontinence, or equipment to ensure their safety around the house. The specific out-of-pocket expenses will vary according to the unique needs of your family member affected by dementia.
- You may need to **adjust your home to enhance its accessibility**. These modifications can include installing ramps for wheelchairs, addressing the need for any stairs lifts, and ensuring the bathroom is safe and easily usable.
- **Care Options for Advancing Dementia**: As dementia progresses, your loved one with dementia may become unable to safely stay alone for any amount of time. In this case, you will need the services of an in-home care nurse, adult daycare, assisted living residence, or residential care facility.

Your health authority, Medicare, or Medicaid may perform a financial evaluation to determine if your loved one qualifies for financial assistance based on their needs.

Alternatively, private care residences are an option, with monthly expenses varying between $1,500 and $5,000 or more, contingent on the required care level and additional services provided.

EVALUATING YOUR RELIANCE ON YOUR JOB'S INCOME FIRST WILL AID YOUR PLANNING AND PREPARATION.

Estimate the cost of caring for your loved one with dementia as accurately as possible.

If necessary, plan a family meeting to address these financial needs. Also, verify if your loved one with dementia has elderly plan insurance.

Creating a strong financial plan means thinking about different situations that might happen and how much they might cost.

Being prepared can really help reduce how much money both you and your loved one with dementia might need to spend.

HOW TO PREPARE FOR A VALUABLE ANNOUNCEMENT MEETING WITH YOUR EMPLOYER

Thoroughly prepare your announcement meeting with your employer to ensure your message is effectively communicated and well-received. You can do this by following the tips below:

- Collect relevant information and supporting documentation.
- Include details about your responsibilities and the type of dementia your loved one has in a concise paragraph.
- Gather information on unpredictable events that you may or may not have faced with some examples. Though speaking about your personal life can be emotional, especially when many difficulties arise, try your best to explain in your documentation that you are planning to live your personal life differently, and that it's highly probable your professional life will also have to adjust.
- Identify potential concerns and solutions.

Try to anticipate any concerns your employer may have, such as the potential impact on your job performance or availability, and to have solutions or alternatives in mind.

You may have to present options like employee programs, flexible hours, and elder care services support.

Take time to choose the option that best suits your situation. Also, be sure to know the different policies your company might offer, including Family and Medical Leave Act (FMLA) policies.

Also, evaluate your vacation time, accrued personal/medical leave, and any carry-over time.

WHAT TO SAY DURING THE MEETING

Come to the meeting with what you wrote about your situation and your plan. Remember that employers prefer accommodating existing employees rather than hiring new ones, as the latter option is more costly and complex.

Share your challenges openly and suggest possible solutions, thus demonstrating your ability to maturely handle your professional and personal life. Doing so also reflects your commitment to maintaining a high level of job performance.

It is helpful to clearly and concisely explain the situation and how it may affect your work. It may also be beneficial to discuss any accommodations or support you might need to continue performing your job effectively.

Ask, ask, and ask for arrangements; you can also prepare a list of resources and present it to your employer, which they can reference in case they need more information.

Doing this will go a long way in showing you have been looking for a workable solution, not just for yourself, but also for your employer.

Thank your employer for his/her openness and readiness to build a system that allows you to function at your best. Note, however, that this first meeting won't be the last.

You will have opportunities to ask for other options if the situation ever changes.

ISSUES YOU MIGHT ENCOUNTER

According to the Alzheimer's Association 2022 Disease Facts and Figures Report, 57% of caregivers had to adjust their work schedules by going in late, leaving early, or taking time off. Additionally, 18% switched from full-time to part-time work, and 16% took a leave of absence.

Some had to make even bigger sacrifices, 9% stopped working entirely, 8% turned down promotions, 7% received warnings about their performance or attendance, 7% lost their benefits, and 6% retired early.

Caregivers, whether caring for elderly relatives or individuals with disabilities, often face many problems when trying to balance their caregiving responsibilities with their jobs.

These problems can lead to significant stress and difficulty maintaining a healthy work-life balance. They can also impact the quality of care provided as a caregiver.

Some of the most common issues caregivers are likely to face with their employers include:

- **Discrimination**: Caregivers may encounter workplace discrimination due to their caregiving responsibilities. Examples of such discrimination include unfair treatment in promotions, terminations, harassment, or pay disparities. Sometimes, employers overlook caregivers for job opportunities precisely due to their caregiving responsibilities.
- Dementia caregivers may **miss opportunities for professional development**, as employers might be less inclined to invest in their training and development, perceiving them as less committed to their jobs. Lack of networking opportunities due to caregiving responsibilities may hinder caregivers from building professional relationships and attending events, potentially limiting their career advancement prospects.

- **Lack of flexibility**: Many caregivers struggle to balance their work and caregiving responsibilities because their employers are unwilling to provide flexible scheduling or other accommodations.
- **Limited access to benefits**: Accessing benefits that could aid in managing their caregiving responsibilities may prove difficult for caregivers. For instance, it might be challenging for caregivers to take time off in order to care for a loved one because many workplaces do not offer paid leave. There may be restrictions or a need to purchase external benefits, including health insurance.
- **Limited support from managers and colleagues**: Managers and colleagues may be unsympathetic or even hostile to caregivers, making it difficult to get the help and support they need from the workplace.
- **Burnout**: As we have studied earlier in this book, caregivers are at high risk of burnout. As a result, they may be overworked, overstressed, and experience isolation and alienation.
- **Financial difficulties**: Caregivers may encounter economic challenges due to their caregiving responsibilities. For example, they may be forced to take unpaid time off or reduce their work hours so they can attend to their loved one's needs. These circumstances can lead to financial hardships, making it difficult to make ends meet.
- **Difficulty balancing work and family**: Caregivers often find it difficult to juggle their work and family responsibilities, which leads to significant stress and difficulty maintaining a healthy work-life balance. They may feel guilty about not being able to spend enough time with their families, or they may think they are neglecting their caregiving responsibilities by focusing on their work.

FIND WAYS TO EXCEL: SET HIGHER GOALS AND ARRANGE PERSONAL CHECKPOINTS TO KEEP YOUR JOB

Dementia caregivers must safeguard their employment amid demanding caregiving duties. Here's how:

- **Be punctual**: Demonstrate reliability and commitment by being on time.
- Demonstrate a **strong work ethic**: Consistently complete tasks to showcase commitment and reliability.
- **Emergency compensation**: Compensate for caregiving emergencies at work by achieving objectives if your pay is results-based or by making up for lost time if your salary is based on hours worked.
- **Maintain open communication**: Keep your employer informed about the impact of caregiving on your work schedule and discuss necessary accommodations.
- **Utilize leave policies**: Take advantage of employer-offered leave policies for caregivers, including unpaid, paid, and flexible scheduling.
- **Prioritize self-care**: Ensure adequate sleep, nutrition, and relaxation for balanced caregiving and work. Refer to Chapter 2 for more information.
- **Professional assistance**: Seek guidance from social workers or geriatric care managers for a tailored care plan. Some employers cover these services in benefit plans, emphasizing their commitment to caregiving support. Remember, you don't have to face it alone; help is available to lighten your load.

Balancing work and caregiving is achievable with effort and planning. By holding yourself to a higher standard, you can reconcile securing your job and providing the best care possible for your loved one with dementia.

BENEFITS AT YOUR WORKPLACE

Many employers value supporting caregiving employees, and can significantly support dementia caregivers through various workplace benefits such as flexible schedules, paid time off, support resources, accommodations, and eldercare assistance programs.

These provisions assist caregivers in balancing their responsibilities and contribute to a more engaged and productive workforce, benefiting caregivers and employers alike. For this reason, many offer time flexibility in corporate benefit plans.

Family caregivers can access flexible time off in various ways. Some companies offer a specified number of paid caregiving days each year, while others provide the option of unpaid leave with job security upon the employee's return to work.

Flexible time off provides several advantages to family caregivers, such as the ability to balance work and caregiving duties, reducing stress, and preventing burnout.

Other workplace accommodations, such as telecommuting and part-time options, may also benefit caregivers.

These policies aid in retaining valuable personnel who might otherwise resign to care for their loved one with dementia. Additionally, they improve morale and employee loyalty by displaying the company's support for its workforce.

Some employers go one step further by offering eldercare assistance programs with resources for caregivers responsible for elderly family members. Caregivers may also receive additional support from their employer, including training programs, support groups, and counseling services that help caregivers better understand dementia, refine care strategies, and develop coping mechanisms.

These programs may also assist in finding care facilities, in-home caregivers, and navigating the healthcare system. In exchange, employers who promote a balance between caregiving duties and job responsibilities benefit from a more engaged and productive workforce.

The dynamic of mutual support enhances employee retention and fosters a reciprocal commitment to organizational success.

HOW TO LOOK FOR A MORE COMPATIBLE JOB

Finding a job compatible with caregiving can be challenging. The pandemic has, however, introduced new possibilities for remote work or hybrid setups (combining remote work and office presence).

It's important to openly communicate your situation to potential employers, sharing your individual circumstances honestly.

Be transparent about your caregiving responsibilities, as many employers are willing to help out, and are open to crafting a suitable schedule to make it happen. Here are a few helpful steps you can take:

- Research employers with a track record of supporting caregivers. Begin by visiting the "People's 2023 List of Companies that Care" on the "Great Place to Work" Institute's website at https://www.greatplacetowork.com/companies-that-care. Then do your due diligence on each company.
- Explore job opportunities with flexible schedules or telecommuting options.
- Use your own personal network to seek opinions and contacts within the targeted companies.

Finding a compatible job may take time, persistence, and patience. But it is worth the price, as it may lead to equilibrium when trying to balance your precious time. The subsequent chart serves as a guide to assist you in determining suitable options based on your work context and caregiving role.

Adapting your job conditions to your caregiver role

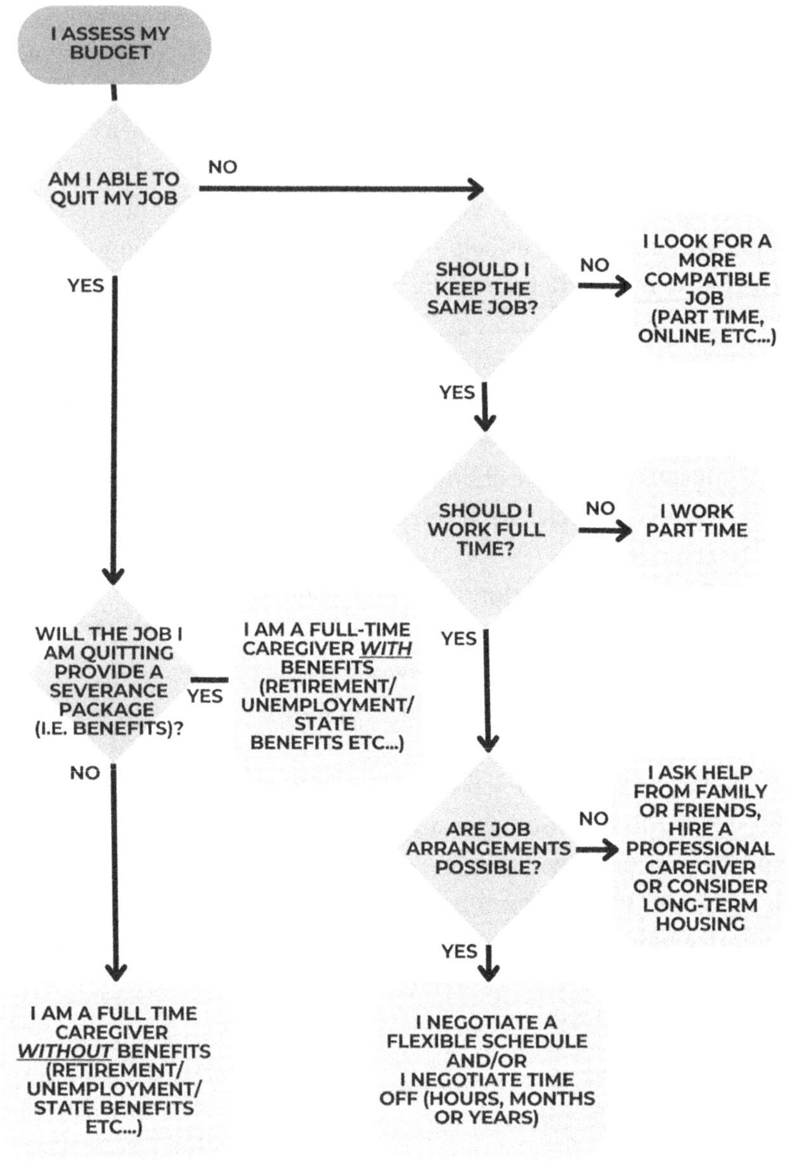

RUNNING A PERSONAL BUSINESS WHILE CARING FOR YOUR LOVED ONE WITH DEMENTIA

Balancing caregiving and entrepreneurship is also demanding, but the following strategies can help:

- **Prioritize and plan**: Create a work schedule focusing on essential tasks (the Eisenhower matrix from Chapter 4 might help). Set specific times for business and caregiving, and streamline the processes.
- **Delegate tasks**: Empower employees, or hire additional staff (if possible), to share business responsibilities.
- **Use technology to boost your productivity**: Stay connected through video conferencing, email, and instant messaging to maintain relationships when physically absent. Also, explore AI tools to automate manual routine tasks that are time-consuming and don't require your analysis, such as taking and organizing meeting notes.
- **Utilize community resources**: Explore respite care, support groups, and in-home services so you can take breaks from caregiving and focus on your business.
- **Seek professional guidance**: Consult business coaches or consultants to guide you in running your business while caring for your loved one with dementia.

Managing the dual roles of caregiving and entrepreneurship demands careful strategies. By applying them, you can maintain your business and provide dedicated care for your loved one with dementia. This approach promotes resilience and success in both caregiving and business endeavors. As we conclude this chapter on balancing caregiving responsibilities with work, it's evident that dementia caregivers face unique challenges that require thoughtful strategies. From securing employment to managing entrepreneurship, the importance of support becomes evident. Moving into the next chapter, we'll delve into the crucial role of a supportive community in the broader context of dementia care.

CHAPTER 9
IT TAKES A VILLAGE TO CARE FOR DEMENTIA

"Sometimes it takes more courage to ask for help than to act alone."

—Ken Petti

As Lovely's dementia progressed, the news of her condition spread within their tight-knit community. Everyone came together to help however they could. The neighbors became like family to Lovely, and offered to help with anything she needed. Jennifer's colleagues at the company she worked for also rallied around her, offering their support and resources.

Even the local support group for dementia caregivers, which Jennifer had joined, reached out to offer help. They became a source of comfort and friendship for both Jennifer and Lovely, providing them with a sense of community and belonging.

Meanwhile, having witnessed Lovely's declining condition during his most recent visit, John resolved to see his mother more frequently to offer increased care and attention, despite his demanding schedule.

The rewarding, yet stressful, nature of his work would no longer deter him from keeping his promise.

Although watching his mom gradually lose her memory and communication abilities was a complicated and emotional process, he wanted to do anything he could to help. So, John discussed with his sister how they could further support their mom, ensuring she didn't feel isolated and anxious. He was also concerned about his sister, feeling she might be overwhelmed by the burden of caring for their mom alone. He didn't know where to turn for support, so he shared his thoughts with Jennifer.

She told her brother about the local support group she had joined, admitting that she hesitated to join at first, but eventually decided to try it. Jennifer went on to tell him how, at the support group, she met other caregivers facing similar challenges, and found comfort in knowing she was not alone. Jennifer further talked about how the support group aimed to maintain pleasant social connections, and how they, along with other individuals within the community, have been reaching out to help her and their mom.

John decided to join Jennifer the next time she attended her support group, and he witnessed the profound challenges his sister faced as a dementia caregiver through what she and others shared during the session. This powerfully emotional experience ignited a passion within him to advocate for the rights of caregivers. When he got back to the big city, John shared his mother's story with everyone he encountered, emphasizing the unique challenges of dementia caregiving, and educated others on the importance of support for both patients and caregivers. His efforts caught the media's attention, and John became a well-known spokesman for dementia awareness. He was invited to speak at conferences and events all over the country, and his message reached thousands of people.

Although she couldn't express it, Lovely continued to find comfort in her daughter Jennifer's care, and appreciated the help and support of family and friends. Jennifer was also grateful for everyone she had met along her caregiving journey. She felt proud of John's advocacy efforts as well. Lovely's condition touched the hearts of many, and showed the power of community. To top it all off, the community discovered that joining forces to assist someone in need fosters stronger connections among people, and has a meaningful impact on the lives of everyone involved.

This chapter emphasizes the importance of having a supportive and loving community around you and your loved one with dementia. While caregivers, often family members, play a primary role in looking after their loved one, dementia care requires a collective effort.

As the chapter unfolds, I will explain how this collaborative approach begins at the "individual scale", where caregivers must navigate the unique challenges of adapting to their loved one's ever-changing needs.

We will then transition to the "community scale", where I'll address the isolation that caregivers often face in our increasingly individualistic era. Here, I will emphasize actionable steps for communities to take toward social engagement and support. Neighbors can become vital allies, offering both social and practical assistance; global initiatives such as *Dementia Friends, USA* attempt to cultivate mutual understanding and support; and dementia-friendly services such as restaurants, cafés, and museums also complement this support network.

Then, at the "organizational scale", I'll talk about how businesses support dementia caregivers with flexible work and counseling, while participating in awareness and fundraising. There are also dementia associations, which educate, support, and advocate for better services, more inclusive policies, and research funding.

On the "societal scale", I will cover how policies influence dementia care by shaping research, access, quality, and economic support. I will insist on the importance of disaster preparedness for dementia caregivers, and recommend toolkits with essential strategies for caregiver readiness.

Finally, on the "global scale", I'll explain how entities, such as the World Health Organization, play a part in this symphony of dementia care. Their influence extends to guidelines, stigma reduction, and advocacy for a comprehensive global response to dementia.

This last chapter will conclude with an expansion from global actions to universal principles of unconditional love and acceptance.

How can we, as humans, improve our quality of support for individuals with dementia and their caregivers? We must be there for each other, sharing stories of life, love, and relationships beyond focusing solely on symptoms or losses. Does this prompt your curiosity? Then, let's rewind and discover the inner layer of the best place on earth: the "Unconditional Love for Dementia Care Global Village."

INDIVIDUAL SCALE

The innermost layer of a global support system for individuals with dementia and their caregivers stands at the individual level. You can't expect your loved one with dementia, siblings, extended family, friends, colleagues, healthcare professionals, neighbors, community, society, and global organizations to change if you don't focus first on embracing your own growth and adaptability to meet the unique needs of your loved one with dementia. Your dedication and compassion will significantly impact their care and well-being. Don't be afraid to fail. Nobody's perfect. Failure leads to learning and adjusting, which is the most beautiful gift you can offer your loved one with dementia each and every day.

COMMUNITY SCALE

Caring for someone with dementia is not solely the responsibility of family and caregivers, but the entire community. A supportive society that values and embraces dementia as a part of the human experience is essential. Yet, according to a 2019 CarersUK report, eight-out-of-ten caregivers feel lonely or isolated, and one-out-of-two would appreciate more understanding from their community.

Okay, but how exactly can the community contribute?

Communities can support persons with dementia and their caregivers by offering social engagement and activities like storytelling and reminiscing groups. For caregivers, these activities may offer respite time. For persons with dementia, they stimulate the brain, provide a sense of purpose, and create connections between their past and the present community they belong to, which is vital when facing memory loss and isolation. Sharing stories and memories helps preserve the bond between individuals with dementia and their community, providing continuity and a connection to the past. Communities can also advocate for dementia awareness and improve care and assistance. Support groups and resources help caregivers learn about the condition, find suitable treatments, and connect with others facing similar challenges. A caring community offers emotional and practical support, enhancing the quality of life for people with dementia.

Neighbors

Neighbors can play a significant role in caring for someone with dementia, forming a supportive community around you and your loved one. They can offer valuable support and a sense of security. One essential role of neighbors in dementia care is providing social support. Your loved one may feel isolated and lonely as their ability to communicate and interact declines. Neighbors can help by visiting them, inviting them over for meals or activities, and keeping them engaged in the community.

"Practical support" from neighbors could be invaluable for you as the caregiver. They could run errands for you and your loved one, provide respite care by watching your loved one for an hour or two, and assist with transportation or occasional meal preparation.

Communicate with neighbors about your loved one's condition, especially symptoms such as wandering, paranoia, and potential vulnerabilities. Neighbors can be a valuable resource if they understand the issues and are willing to help. Don't hesitate to seek assistance from them if they are supportive. If they turn out to be more problematic than helpful, ensure there's a backup available to care for your loved one with dementia. A robust and reliable support system provides the best care possible.

Dementia Friends

The "Dementia Friends" program is a valuable initiative to increase understanding and support for individuals with dementia. Launched by the Alzheimer's Society of the UK in 2013, it has expanded to other countries, including the US. To become a "Dementia Friend", extended family, friends, neighbors, or others can attend a session or take an online course to learn about dementia's impact on people's lives. These sessions provide helpful tips on communication and interaction with individuals with dementia.

"Dementia Friends" are compassionate and supportive individuals who understand the challenges faced by people with dementia and their caregivers. They offer patience, kindness, and assistance when needed, and share knowledge about dementia with others to increase awareness. The program has created a more compassionate society, reduced stigma, and fostered inclusivity for people with dementia in their communities. It's a valuable resource that promotes understanding and actively empowers individuals to support those with dementia.

Services Around You

Various services are available to support people living with dementia and their caregivers. These services provide the necessary care and support throughout your loved one's journey. We will explore some of these services now:

- **A dementia-friendly restaurant** is a restaurant that has made specific adjustments to its environment, staff training, and menu options to provide a welcoming and comfortable experience for people living with dementia and their caregivers. One of the main features of a dementia-friendly restaurant is its environment, which includes good lighting, clear signage, and non-slip flooring to reduce the risk of accidents and injuries. The restaurant may also provide comfortable seating and a quiet and calming atmosphere. The staff understands dementia and how it affects people and is trained to offer helpful and respectful service. "Purple tables" are another feature of eateries catering to people with dementia. These tables are designated as a safe space for people living with dementia because they are easy to spot and are in a quiet area of the restaurant, thereby soothing people with dementia who may become confused or disoriented in a noisy environment. The purple also serves as a visual cue for staff, indicating that the people sitting at the table may need extra assistance or verbal cues to help with food choices.

- **A dementia-friendly café** is a community group that allows people with dementia and their caregivers to connect with others who share their circumstances. It usually meets in a nearby public location, such as a church hall or community center. It is a welcoming and understanding group, typically led by a health or social care professional. However, it may occasionally be hosted by a nearby charity or volunteers specially trained to assist persons with dementia. Dementia-friendly cafes are a great place to discuss your loved one's dementia diagnosis with a trained professional who can answer your questions and share experiences with others on a similar journey. You can also make new friends, boosting your confidence and self-esteem. These cafes offer a sense of normalcy and familiarity, allowing people with dementia to keep their independence and enjoy a few of the activities they loved before their diagnosis. It's a supportive and welcoming environment that can positively impact your loved one's life.
- **Dementia-friendly museums** make specific adjustments to their environment, staff training, and exhibits to accommodate the unique needs of dementia patients. Dementia-friendly museums provide a stimulating, engaging environment that promotes cognitive and social interaction. They offer educational and cultural activities to stimulate cognitive function and reduce feelings of isolation and loneliness. They provide opportunities to reminisce and share experiences, which can be therapeutic and reinforce a sense of identity.

Now that we've covered ways the community can get involved in supporting you and your loved one with dementia, let's continue our exploration at the organizational level.

ORGANIZATIONAL SCALE

At the organizational level, the role of businesses and associations is key.

Companies

Businesses can contribute significantly by offering various systems and services tailored to meet the unique needs of individuals with dementia and their families. These contributions are vital in enhancing their quality of life. They include:

- Providing **support for employees** who have a family member with dementia: offering flexible work arrangements, counseling services, and educational resources.
- **Raising funds** for charities, volunteering, or organizing events to raise awareness of dementia and its effects on families and communities. These can all be done in collaboration with neighborhood organizations.
- **Developing products or services** to assist in caring for individuals with dementia, such as assistive technology, specialized clothing, or memory aids.

Associations

Dementia associations have a variety of roles in the care of dementia patients, which include:

- Providing **information and resources** to individuals with dementia, their caregivers, and families.
- Offering **support groups and counseling services**.
- **Advocating** for the rights and needs of individuals with dementia: This can include lobbying for better access to services, more funding for research, and more inclusive and dementia-friendly policies.
- **Financing research** to help improve our understanding of dementia and the management of symptoms until a cure is found.

- **Offering respite** care and support for caregivers.

Let's now move on to the societal scale.

SOCIETAL SCALE

At the societal scale, government policies, regulations, and laws can significantly impact the care and support given to individuals with dementia, both positively and negatively. How?

- Government **policies and regulations** can affect the funding for research, healthcare, and support services for individuals with dementia. Policies and regulations can lessen the economic burden of dementia on people with dementia and their caregivers through government-funded healthcare, social security, and disability benefits, caregiver support programs, long-term care insurance, or tax benefits and deductions.
- **Access** to care: Laws and regulations can determine the type and quality of care and support services available to individuals with dementia.
- **Quality of care**: Policies and regulations can set standards for the quality of care provided to individuals with dementia, including requirements for training and accreditation of healthcare professionals.
- **Discrimination**: Laws and regulations can prohibit discrimination against individuals with dementia, ensuring they have the same rights and opportunities as others.

"Zoom in" on Environmental Considerations and Disaster Preparedness

In today's unpredictable world, preparing for potential environmental disasters is crucial, especially for the most vulnerable individuals. The intensification of extreme weather events, rising sea levels, and volatile environmental shifts necessitate a proactive approach to preparing for and mitigating the risks of such calamities.

In 2010, a study done by Dosa and team, published in the *Disaster Medicine and Public Health Preparedness* journal revealed a significant increase in mortality, hospitalization, and functional decline among nursing facility residents during Hurricane Katrina. It is not a stretch to extend this finding to seniors, particularly those with dementia, such as your loved one.

Why share this information? Not to dwell on the negative, but to raise awareness among caregivers like you about the potential impact natural disasters can have on your loved one with dementia, especially with the heightened threat of global warming looming just overhead. While community and societal involvement in environmental matters is essential, having a well-thought-out emergency plan for you and your loved one with dementia is even more critical.

The preparation can be challenging though, especially as individuals with dementia may struggle to understand and respond appropriately to emergency circumstances. Regarding this matter, the US Administration on Aging actually financed a project on disaster preparedness that was developed by the Alzheimer's Association. The objective is to summarize key action plans for states, such as coordinating with emergency management offices and educating the aging population. At the same time, caregivers are advised to create personal disaster plans and prepare accordingly.

To help with this, the National Alzheimer's and Dementia Resource Center (NADRC) provides an "Emergency Preparedness Toolkit for People Living with Dementia," updated in April 2022. It equips caregivers with essential information to address specific challenges that may arise during a disaster using four toolkits with very well thought-out checklists.

The first toolkit focuses on communication, offering comprehensive strategies for understanding and supporting individuals with dementia. It addresses behavioral challenges, sleep management, and emotional well-being during crises. Additionally, it emphasizes maintaining routines and ensuring proper nutrition and hydration.

The second toolkit provides a tailored emergency supply checklist for dementia caregivers.

The third toolkit guides caregivers on essential contact information, including numbers for FEMA, the Red Cross, and Disaster Recovery Centers.

And the last toolkit helps caregivers track medical conditions, specific care needs, and life preferences, such as daily routines and hobbies.

To wrap up the societal section, let's review what we've covered so far. We've explored how government policies shape dementia care at the social level, and emphasized the importance of disaster preparedness.

Remember to get those toolkits. They will equip you to face challenges that may arise during unexpected disasters.

Next, as we transition to the global scale, let's talk about the pivotal role of entities like the World Health Organization in orchestrating a comprehensive global response to dementia.

GLOBAL SCALE

The World Health Organization (WHO) has been significantly shaping the global response to dementia care. Through initiatives like the "Global Status Report on the Public Health Response to Dementia", the WHO sets guidelines, raises awareness, reduces stigma, and advocates for worldwide action to enhance dementia care and support. As per the WHO's "Global Status Report on the Public Health Response to Dementia," approximately one-fourth of nations globally possess a national policy, strategy, or plan supporting dementia patients and their families. Some of these initiatives, notably in Europe, are either reaching conclusion or have already expired, demonstrating the need for governments to recommit.

The World Health Organization has identified dementia as a significant global health concern and has implemented a strategic plan effective until 2025, known as the "Global Action Plan on the Public Health Response to Dementia." This comprehensive program encompasses various facets, including raising public awareness, reducing risk factors, improving care, and advancing research initiatives. Monitoring progress, the Global Dementia Observatory (GDO) collects data on key indicators, while the Knowledge Exchange Platform facilitates the sharing of best practices, fostering international collaboration and knowledge dissemination.

The WHO influences dementia care in many other ways as well, including:

- Setting **guidelines and standards** for diagnosing, treating, and caring for individuals with dementia. These guidelines help ensure that care is provided consistently and in a high-quality manner worldwide.
- **Raising awareness and reducing stigma**: The WHO works to raise awareness of dementia and its impact on individuals, families, and communities, and looks for ways to reduce the stigma associated with the condition.
- **Advocating for global action**: The WHO advocates for global action on dementia, including increased funding for research and support services, while developing policies and laws that promote the rights and needs of individuals with dementia.

In 2021, the World Health Organization released the "Towards a Dementia-Inclusive Society" toolkit, guiding countries to empower individuals with dementia within their communities. This toolkit advocates for values that convey universal principles such as tolerance, inclusiveness, and unconditional love. The WHO's toolkit provides a practical answer to the question raised in the introduction of this chapter: "How can we, as humans, improve our quality of support for individuals with dementia and their caregivers?"

A dementia-inclusive society ensures active engagement and inclusion of individuals with dementia and their caregivers within the community. It affords them respect, freedom, dignity, equality, and an improved quality of life. In such a society, they are encouraged to live independently, without stigma, discrimination, exploitation, violence, or abuse.

Freedom is about giving individuals with dementia and their caregivers choices. They get to decide whether they want to be known as someone with dementia or not. They get to decide if they want to participate in different activities. We must create a dementia-friendly environment to give them this free choice. Education is the key to making sure our society is genuinely inclusive towards them. It means teaching our communities, governments, medical professionals, teachers, and students about dementia, starting when we're young. Everyone wants to feel accepted and loved for who they are, not for what they can, cannot, or can no longer do.

Initiatives like *The Agency for Integrated Care* (AIC), supported by the Ministry of Health (MOH) in Singapore, are an inspirational example of joint efforts toward demystifying dementia. Dementia-Friendly Communities (DFCs) are in different neighborhoods nationwide to create a "place where persons with dementia and their caregivers can live as independently as possible while feeling safe, loved, comfortable, and respected." In these communities, people learn about dementia, and those with dementia and their families are supported in ways that allow them to live well.

The DFCs follow the "3Es" approach: Engage, Empower, and Enable. They educate the community; empower people with dementia and caregivers, offering them assistance, autonomy, and choice; and enhance technology and infrastructure to support them. There are already ten DFCs in Singapore, and the goal is to build more, ensuring a caring and inclusive society for those with dementia and their caregivers. Initiatives like these are prime examples to emulate in creating a more inclusive, dementia-friendly world.

HELLO, INCREDIBLE CAREGIVER!
I NEED YOUR HELP!

Is this information helping you? If so, please leave a review. Your thoughts and opinions hold immense value in shaping the choices of others.

To review and rate my book, follow these easy steps:

1. Open your phone's camera.
2. Point it at the QR code below to reveal a link.
3. Click the link to review and rate my book.

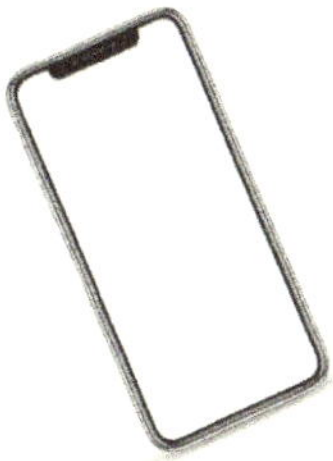

Thank you so much!

ONLY 60 SECONDS CAN MAKE A BIG DIFFERENCE FOR OTHER CAREGIVERS

CONCLUSION

"You can't calm the storm, so stop trying. What you can do is calm yourself. The storm will pass."

—Timber Hawkeye

Caring for a loved one with dementia is a challenging and emotional journey. Despite the difficulties, it is essential to understand the different stages of dementia and be familiar with the common symptoms that may occur during each stage. This will enhance your grasp of your loved one's behavior, enabling you to respond appropriately with patience, compassion, and self-understanding. By taking care of yourself along this path, you will find the strength and resilience needed to provide the best care possible for your loved one with dementia.

Effective communication is critical in caring for your loved one with dementia. Speak, use simple language, and avoid distractions. It is also helpful to validate your loved one's feelings and to avoid correcting them if they have a mistaken perception.

Create a safe and secure environment. Ensure your loved one's surroundings are familiar and comfortable. Ensure they receive sufficient supervision during their activities of daily living, such as bathing and dressing, to prevent accidents.

Regarding financial and legal matters, such as Power of Attorney, dealing with them early in the dementia care journey (preferably right after the diagnosis), can make a significant difference. Keeping track of all expenses and seeking guidance from a Medicaid/Medicare specialist can help you identify available financial assistance. Make these arrangements to secure a smoother caregiving experience and focus more on cherishing the precious moments you have with your loved one.

Ensure your loved one receives sufficient stimulation through activities they enjoy, such as exercise, music, art, gardening, etc. These provide a sense of purpose and enjoyment that can play a significant role in keeping your loved one fulfilled until the end. Maintaining contact with friends and family is an excellent way to preserve your loved one's communication and social skills, and keep them active in their community.

Finally, as you embark on this complex journey, know that resources are available to help you, and you're not alone as a caregiver. Also, know that emotions are among the most resilient abilities of the brain; and, no matter the stage your loved one is in, you can use this emotional resilience to connect with your loved one with dementia in a positive and meaningful way.

Professionals understand how to harness and teach strategies to utilize your loved one's remaining abilities. One efficient approach in this regard is music therapy. Music is directly wired to your loved one's emotional centers in the brain while stimulating other capabilities, such as movement, language, memory, and auditory sense. Music may well allow you to connect with your loved one with dementia in a profound and fulfilling way, even in the later stages. Thus, would you like my next book to teach you how to purposefully use music to stimulate and connect with your loved one with dementia? Let me know by providing your answer in this form. Scan the QR code to access it.

Caregiving is indeed a challenging and demanding task. But it is also an opportunity to show love and compassion to your loved one with dementia when they need it the most. The positive facets of dementia caregiving are extensive, encompassing a sense of personal achievement, a mutually enriching relationship with your loved one, enhanced family unity, and an amplified sense of personal development and life purpose. These findings were articulated in a comprehensive review conducted by Doris Yu and her research team in 2018.

By understanding the needs of your loved one with dementia and utilizing available resources, you can provide the best possible care. You don't need to go it alone. Support groups, respite care, home care assistance, and professional counseling are valuable resources that can help you reduce the stress and burden of caregiving.

Remember to take one day at a time and seek help when needed. I know you're already achieving wonderful results with your loved one with dementia, and you will continue to grow as a dementia caregiver and as a human being.

I wish you continued meaningful and memorable moments with your loved one with dementia, authentic connections with them and their helpers amidst the most challenging symptoms, and countless blessings on your caregiving journey!

With love,

Stéphane Suppervielle

P.S: Join our **Practical Dementia Caregiver Support Group** on Facebook. Visit **soaring-eagle.com/facebook**

BIBLIOGRAPHY

5 Challenges and benefits of joining a dementia support group. (2017, June 20). Samvedna Care. https://www.samvednacare.com/blog/5-challenges-and-benefits-of-joining-a-dementia-support-group/

7 Ways to Build a Strong Relationship with Your Doctor. (2022, September 2). Scripps Health. https://www.scripps.org/news_items/5394-7-ways-to-build-a-strong-relationship-with-your-doctor

20 self-care activities you can do in 10 minutes or less. (2023). Confident Life. https://www.-confidentlife.com.au/20-quick-self-care-activities-can-10-mins-less/

23 best caregiver support groups online and in-person. (2021, March 16). A Place for Mom. https://www.aplaceformom.com/caregiver-resources/articles/caregiver-support-groups

Activities for people with dementia: 30 expert tips for daily activities and routines. (2023, October 24). Careforth. https://careforth.com/blog/activities-for-dementia-patients-50-tips-and-ideas-to-keep-patients-with-dementia-engaged/

Abrams, B. (2015). Humanistic approaches. In B. L. Wheeler (Ed.), *Music therapy handbook* (pp. 148-160). Guilford Press.

Agronin, M. E. (2015). *The dementia caregiver: A Guide to Caring for Someone with Alzheimer's Disease and Other Neurocognitive Disorders.* Rowman & Littlefield.

AGS - Geriatrics Healthcare Professionals. (2018, October 10). *Setting Personal Goals for Dementia Care.* Health in Aging. https://www.healthinaging.org/blog/setting-personal-goals-for-dementia-care/

AIC Singapore. (June 2022). *A Caregiver's Guide to Avoid Burnout.* https://www.aic.sg/resources/Documents/Brochures/Caregiving%20Support/Caregiver%20Burnout%20Guide%20EN.pdf

Almeida, D., & Marinho, G. (2021). 505 - Reversible Dementia caused by Hypothyroidism – a case report. *International Psychogeriatrics, 33*(S1), 58. https://doi.org/10.1017/s1041610221002003

Alzheimer's and related dementias - American Association for Geriatric Psychiatry. (2023). American Association for Geriatric Psychiatry. https://www.aagponline.org/index.php?src=gendocs&ref=Dementia_factsheet&category=Foundation.

Alzheimer's Association. (2019a). *Caregiver stress.* https://www.alz.org/help-support/caregiving/caregiver-health/caregiver-stress

Alzheimer's Association. (2019b). *Communication and Alzheimer's.* https://www.alz.org/help-support/caregiving/daily-care/communications

Alzheimer's Association. (2019c). *Event search.* https://www.alz.org/events/event_search?etid=2&cid=0

Alzheimer's Association. (2019d). *Medical tests.* https://www.alz.org/alzheimers-dementia/diagnosis/medical_tests

Alzheimer's Association. (2019e). *Visiting your doctor.* https://www.alz.org/alzheimers-dementia/diagnosis/visiting-your-doctor

Alzheimer's Association. (2022). *Stages of Alzheimer's*. https://www.alz.org/alzheimers-dementia/stages

Alzheimer's Association. (2023a). 2023 Alzheimer's disease facts and figures. https://www.alz.org/media/Documents/alzheimers-facts-and-figures.pdf

Alzheimer's Association. (2023b). *Alzheimer's disease facts and figures*. https://www.alz.org/alzheimers-dementia/facts-figures

Alzheimer's Association. (2023c). *Financial planning*. https://www.alz.org/help-support/i-have-alz/plan-for-your-future/financial_planning

Alzheimer's Society. (2019, August 02). *How to offer help to someone with dementia who doesn't want it*. https://www.alzheimers.org.uk/blog/how-offer-help-someone-dementia-who-doesnt-want-it

Alzheimer's Society. (2021a, February 24). *The middle stage of dementia*. https://www.alzheimers.org.uk/about-dementia/symptoms-and-diagnosis/how-dementia-progresses/middle-stage-dementia

Alzheimer's Society. (2021b, June 18). *The later stage of dementia*. https://www.alzheimers.org.uk/about-dementia/symptoms-and-diagnosis/how-dementia-progresses/later-stages-dementia

Alzheimer's Society. (2022, June 21). *What is vascular dementia?* https://www.alzheimers.org.uk/about-dementia/types-dementia/vascular-dementia

Alzheimer's Society. (2023a, April 13). *Risk factors for Alzheimer's disease*. https://www.alzheimers.org.uk/about-dementia/types-dementia/who-gets-alzheimers-disease#content-start

Alzheimer's Society. (2023b, August 1). *How physical and sensory difficulties can affect eating*. https://www.alzheimers.org.uk/get-support/daily-living/eating-physical-sensory-difficulties#:

Alzheimer Society of Canada. (2016). *Caregiver stress assessment checklist*. https://alzheimer.ca/sites/default/files/documents/Caregiver-stress-assessment-checklist--Alzheimer-Society.pdf

Alzheimer Society of Canada. (2019a). *Ambiguous loss and grief in dementia*. https://alzheimer.ca/sites/default/files/documents/ambiguous-loss-and-grief_for-individuals-and-families.pdf

Alzheimer Society of Canada. (2019b). *The role of friends and family getting a diagnosis*. https://alzheimer.ca/sites/default/files/documents/alzheimers-disease_getting-a-diagnosis_0.pdf

Alzheimer Society of Canada. (2022). *Reducing caregiver stress*. https://alzheimer.ca/en/help-support/im-caring-person-living-dementia/looking-after-yourself/reducing-caregiver-stress#10_warning_signs_of_stress

Alzheimer Society of Canada. (2023a). *Getting a diagnosis toolkit*. https://alzheimer.ca/sites/default/files/documents/getting-a-diagnosis-toolkit.pdf

Alzheimer Society of Canada. (2023b). *The differences between normal aging and dementia*. https://alzheimer.ca/en/about-dementia/do-i-have-dementia/differences-between-normal-aging-dementia

Blandin, K., & Pepin, R. (2016). Dementia grief: A theoretical model of a unique grief experience. *Dementia, 16*(1), 67–78. https://doi.org/10.1177/1471301215581081

Boso, M., Politi, P., Barale, F., & Enzo, E. (2006). Neurophysiology and neurobiology of the musical experience. *Functional neurology, 21*(4), 187-191. https://pubmed.ncbi.nlm.nih.gov/17367577/

Boss, P. (2000). *Ambiguous loss: Learning to live with unresolved grief.* Harvard University Press.

Brodaty, H., & Donkin, M. (2009). Family caregivers of people with dementia. *Dialogues in Clinical Neuroscience, 11*(2), 217–228. https://doi.org/10.31887/dcns.2009.11.2/hbrodaty

Budson, A. E. (2022, January 20). *Why are women more likely to develop Alzheimer's disease?* https://www.health.harvard.edu/blog/why-are-women-more-likely-to-develop-alzheimers-disease-202201202672#:

Burke, R. (2019, August 21). *How to stay positive as a dementia caregiver: 25 affirmations.* https://www.linkedin.com/pulse/how-stay-positive-dementia-caregiver-25-affirmations-rosanne-burke

Burns, A., Gallagley, A., Byrne, J. (2004, March 1). *Delirium.* Journal of Neurology, Neurosurgery & Psychiatry. https://jnnp.bmj.com/content/75/3/362

Bursack, C. B. (2022, April 25). *Should you quit your job to care for your elderly parent?* Should I Quit My Job To Take Care of My Elderly Parents? - AgingCare.com. https://www.agingcare.com/articles/should-you-quit-your-job-to-care-for-your-elderly-parent-150227.htm

Carbone, J. T., Dell, N. A., Issa, M., & Watkins, M. A. (2022). Associations between allostatic load and posttraumatic stress disorder: A scoping review. *Health & Social Work, 47*(2), 132-142. https://doi.org/10.1093/hsw/hlac001

CarersUK. (2019). Facts about Carers (rep.). https://www.carersuk.org/news/10-facts-about-loneliness-and-caring-in-the-uk-for-loneliness-awareness-week/#_ftn2.

Carescout. (2021). Genworth Cost of Care Survey. Genworth. https://www.genworth.com/aging-and-you/finances/cost-of-care.html

Catastrophic reactions. (n.d.). Homewatch CareGivers. https://www.homewatchcaregivers.com/dementia/symptoms/catastrophic-reactions

Cations, M., Low, L.-F., Blair, A., & Koder, D. (2020, December). *Psychological therapy for people with dementia.* APS. https://psychology.org.au/for-members/publications/inpsych/2020/dec-jan-issue-6/psychological-therapy-for-people-with-dementia

Coates, C. (2023, July 1). *How museums are reaching out to people with dementia.* MuseumNext. https://www.museumnext.com/article/designing-museum-programmes-for-people-with-dementia/

Cognitive Assessment & Care Plan Services. (n.d.). MediCare. https://www.medicare.gov/coverage/cognitive-assessment-care-plan-services

Companies that Care. (2023). PEOPLE | Great Place to Work. https://www.greatplacetowork.com/best-workplaces/companies-that-care/2023

Crowe, A. (2022, March 10). *Amid a Geriatrician Shortage, Nurses Answer the Call.* https://scienceofcaring.ucsf.edu/education/amid-geriatrician-shortage-nurses-answer-call

Cuddy, L. L., & Duffin, J. (2005). Music, memory, and alzheimer's disease: Is music recognition spared in dementia, and how can it be assessed? *Medical Hypotheses, 64*(2), 229-235. https://doi.org/10.1016/j.mehy.2004.09.005

Degges-White, S. (2015, March 23). *The 13 essential traits of good friends.* Psychology Today.

https://www.psychologytoday.com/ca/blog/lifetime-connections/201503/the-13-essential-traits-good-friends

Delirium vs. dementia – understanding the differences. (2023, September 27). BetterHelp. https://www.betterhelp.com/advice/dementia/delirium-vs-dementia-understanding-the-differences/

Dementia & foul language – why some people with dementia develop problems with swearing. (2023). Dementia Care Central. https://www.dementiacarecentral.com/video/swearing/

Dementia friends. (2022, February 24). Alzheimer's Orange County. https://www.alzoc.org/dementia-friends/

Discover Your Love Language - 5 Love Languages. (2023). Northfield Publishing. https://5lovelanguages.com/

Dosa, D., Feng, Z., Hyer, K., Brown, L. M., Thomas, K., & Mor, V. (2010). Effects of Hurricane Katrina on nursing facility resident mortality, hospitalization, and functional decline. *Disaster Medicine and Public Health Preparedness,* 4(S1). https://doi.org/10.1001/dmp.2010.11

Do's and Don'ts of communication and dementia. (2023, January 20). Alzheimer's San Diego. https://www.alzsd.org/dos-and-donts-of-compassionate-communication-dementia/

Do's and don'ts of dementia care. (2017, June 5). Friendship Haven. https://www.friendshiphaven.org/dos-and-donts-of-dementia-care

Eimer, W. A., Vijaya Kumar, D. K., Navalpur Shanmugam, N. K., Rodriguez, A. S., Mitchell, T., Washicosky, K. J., György, B., Breakefield, X. O., Tanzi, R. E., & Moir, R. D. (2018). Alzheimer's disease-associated β-amyloid is rapidly seeded by Herpesviridae to protect against brain infection. *Neuron, 99*(1). https://doi.org/10.1016/j.neuron.2018.06.030

Endsjo, A. (2016, November 20). *Dementia: What part of the brain is under attack?* Permobil. https://hub.permobil.com/blog/dementia-what-part-of-the-brain-is-under-attack

Feurich, V. (2021, January 12). 5 Tips for Communicating Better When Dementia Is Involved. *Positive Approach to Care.* https://teepasnow.com/blog/teepa_snow_tips_-for_communicating_better/

Fink, J. L. W. (2022, February 15). *How dementia kills.* Healthgrades. https://www.healthgrades.com/right-care/dementia/how-dementia-kills

Fogel, M. (2016). Supporting families of people living with dementia. *Social Work Today, 16*(6), 14–17. https://www.socialworktoday.com/archive/111516p14.shtml

Gallego-Alberto, L., Losada, A., Cabrera, I., Romero-Moreno, R., Pérez-Miguel, A., Pedroso-Chaparro, M. D., & Márquez-González, M. (2020, June 4). "I feel guilty". Exploring guilt-related dynamics in family caregivers of people with dementia. *Clinical Gerontologist, 45*(5), 1294–1303. https://doi.org/10.1080/07317115.2020.1769244

García-Valverde, E., Badia, M., Orgaz, M. B., & Gónzalez-Ingelmo, E. (2019). The influence of songwriting on quality of life of family caregivers of people with dementia: An exploratory study. *Nordic Journal of Music Therapy, 29*(1), 4–19. https://doi.org/10.1080/08098131.2019.1630666

Geriatrics still failing to attract new doctors. (2018, February 27). Modern Healthcare. https://www.modernhealthcare.com/article/20180227/NEWS/180229926/geriatrics-still-failing-to-attract-new-doctors

Good, M. (2017, March 13). *When a neighbor with dementia wanders and becomes lost.* Together in This. https://togetherinthis.com/neighbor-wanders/

Gore, R. L., Vardy, E. R., & O'Brien, J. T. (2014). Delirium and dementia with Lewy bodies: Distinct diagnoses or part of the same spectrum? *Journal of Neurology, Neurosurgery & Psychiatry, 86*(1), 50–59. https://doi.org/10.1136/jnnp-2013-306389

Hardy, D. (2022). *The compound effect.* John Murray Learning.

Hornby, L. (n.d.). *Candy to support hydration: Official website.* Jelly Drops USA. https://www.jellydrops.us/

Howley, E. K. (2018, April 13). *5 questions to ask during your first visit with a geriatrician.* U.S. News. https://health.usnews.com/health-care/patient-advice/articles/2018-04-13/5-questions-to-ask-during-your-first-visit-with-a-geriatrician

Howley, E. K. (2022, July 6). *Which doctor should I see for dementia.* U.S. News. https://health.usnews.com/health-care/patient-advice/which-doctor-should-i-see-for-dementia-and-cognitive-decline

Johns Hopkins Medicine. (2021, November 23). *Specialists in aging: Do you need a geriatrician?* https://www.hopkinsmedicine.org/health/wellness-and-prevention/specialists-in-aging-do-you-need-a-geriatrician

Johns Hopkins Medicine. (2022, February 8). *Facing dementia in the family.* https://www.hopkinsmedicine.org/health/conditions-and-diseases/dementia/facing-dementia-in-the-family

Juster, R.-P., McEwen, B. S., & Lupien, S. J. (2010, September). Allostatic load biomarkers of chronic stress and impact on health and cognition. *Neuroscience & Biobehavioral Reviews, 35*(1), 2–16. https://doi.org/10.1016/j.neubiorev.2009.10.002

Känel, R., Dimsdale, J. E., Patterson, T. L., & Grant, I. (2003, August 1). Acute procoagulant stress response as a dynamic measure of allostatic load in alzheimer caregivers. *Annals of Behavioral Medicine, 26*(1), 42–48. https://doi.org/10.1207/s15324796abm2601_06

Kinoshita, M. (2019, July). Addressing dementia: The roles played by businesses. Mitsui & Co., Ltd. https://www.mitsui.com/mgssi/en/report/detail/__icsFiles/afieldfile/2019/08/20/1907t_kinoshita_e_2.pdf

Klein, S. L., & Flanagan, K. L. (2016, August 22). Sex differences in immune responses. *Nature Reviews Immunology, 16*(10), 626–638. https://doi.org/10.1038/nri.2016.90

Leonard, J. (2021, March 4). *How to let go of the past.* Medical News Today. https://www.medicalnewstoday.com/articles/how-to-let-go-of-the-past

Los Angeles County Department of Public Health. (2022). *Supporting people with dementia: A resource guide for social workers.* Healthy Brain LA Program. Los Angeles, CA. http://publichealth.lacounty.gov/seniorhealth/docs/Supporting%20People%20with%20Dementia-A%20Resource%20Guide%20for%20Social%20Workers-Dec2022.pdf

Losada, A., Márquez-González, M., Peñacoba, C., & Romero-Moreno, R. (2010, February 22). *Development and validation of the caregiver guilt questionnaire: International psychogeriatrics.* Cambridge Core. https://www.cambridge.org/core/journals/international-psychogeriatrics/article/abs/development-and-validation-of-the-caregiver-guilt-questionnaire/E07CAA3C7A2E6D8761085ED3B7452B5A

Mace, N. L., & Rabins, P. V. (2017). *The 36-hour day: A family guide to caring for people who have alzheimer disease, related dementias, and memory loss.* Johns Hopkins University Press.

Mayo Foundation for Medical Education and Research. (2023, August 30). *Dementia.* Mayo Clinic. https://www.mayoclinic.org/diseases-conditions/dementia/symptoms-causes/syc-20352013

Michas, F. (2022). Alzheimer-dementia caregivers with work-related changes U.S. 2017. Statista. https://www.statista.com/statistics/452952/workrelated-changes-in-caregivers-for-alzheimers-and-dementia-patients-in-the-us

Mograbi, D. C., Huntley, J., & Critchley, H. (2021, November 24). Self-awareness in dementia: A taxonomy of processes, overview of findings, and integrative framework. *Current Neurology and Neuroscience Reports, 21*(12). https://doi.org/10.1007/s11910-021-01155-6

National Alzheimer's and Dementia Resource Center. (2018, September 26). *NADRC Resource: Emergency Preparedness Toolkit for People Living with Dementia.* Administration for Community Living. https://nadrc.acl.gov/details?search1=151

National Institutes of Health. (2017a, May 16). *What happens to the brain in alzheimer's disease?* National Institute on Aging. https://www.nia.nih.gov/health/what-happens-brain-alzheimers-disease

National Institutes of Health. (2017b, May 17). *Tips for coping with sundowning.* National Institute on Aging. https://www.nia.nih.gov/health/alzheimers-changes-behavior-and-communication/tips-coping-sundowning

National Institutes of Health. (2021, July 30). *What are frontotemporal disorders? Causes, symptoms, and treatment.* National Institute on Aging. https://www.nia.nih.gov/health/what-are-frontotemporal-disorders

Navigating family dynamics when caring for aging parents: An interview with Francine Russo. (2014, June 11). Changing the Way the World Ages. http://changingthewaytheworldages.com/navigating-family-dynamics-when-caring-for-aging-parents-an-interview-with-francine-russo/

Neurologists: Do seniors with Alzheimer's need one? (2021, October 13). *Five Star Senior Living.* https://www.fivestarseniorliving.com/blog/neurologists-do-seniors-with-alzheimers-need-one

N.U.T.S. - Understanding stress. (2015, January 14). Heart-Mind Online. https://heartmindonline.org/resources/nuts-understanding-stress

Onyike, C. U. (2016, April 22). *Psychiatric aspects of dementia.* National Library of Medicine. https://www.ncbi.nlm.nih.gov/pmc/articles/PMC5390928/

Realpharmaneeds. (2021, September 22). Alzheimer!! don't forget to read this! [Blog post]. *Dailygram.* https://dailygram.com/blog/989124/alzheimer-dont-forget-to-read-this/

Reisberg, B., Ferris, S. H., De Leon, M. J., & Crook, T. (1982). The global deterioration scale for assessment of primary degenerative dementia. American Journal of Psychiatry, 139(9), 1136–1139. https://doi.org/10.1176/ajp.139.9.1136

Reitman Centre Team. (2020, May 21). *When friends and family don't understand the impact of dementia caregiving.* Sinai Health. https://www.dementiacarers.ca/when-friends-and-family-dont-understand-the-impact-of-dementia-caregiving/

Reuben, D. B., & Fulmer, T. (2021, February 11). Nurse practitioners and dementia care: A perfect fit. *The American Journal of Geriatric Psychiatry, 29*(6), 527–529. https://doi.org/10.1016/j.jagp.2021.02.040

Richardson, S., Lawson, R. A., Price, A., & Taylor, J.-P. (2022, October 25). Challenges in diagnosis and management of delirium in lewy body disease. *Acta Psychiatrica Scandinavica, 147*(5), 475–480. https://doi.org/10.1111/acps.13514

Richardson, T. J., Lee, S. J., Berg-Weger, M., & Grossberg, G. T. (2013, July 15). Caregiver health: Health of caregivers of alzheimer's and other dementia patients. *Current Psychiatry Reports, 15*(7). https://doi.org/10.1007/s11920-013-0367-2

Rio, R. (2018). A community-based music therapy support group for people with alzheimer's disease and their caregivers: A sustainable partnership model. *Frontiers in Medicine, 5*. https://doi.org/10.3389/fmed.2018.00293

Rogers, C. R. (1959). A theory of therapy, personality, and interpersonal relationships: As developed in the client-centered framework. In S. Koch (Ed.), *Psychology: A Study of a Science. Formulations of the Person and the Social Context* (Vol. 3, pp. 184-256). New York: McGraw Hill.

Rogers, N. (2013). Person-centred expressive arts therapy: Connecting body, mind, and spirit. In M. Cooper, C. O'Hara, P. F. Schmid, & A. C. Bohart (Eds.), *The Handbook of Person-Centred Psychotherapy & Counselling* (2nd ed., pp. 237–247). London: Palgrave Macmillan.

Rolvsjord, R. (2015, June 9). Resource-oriented perspectives in music therapy. *Oxford Handbooks Online*. https://doi.org/10.1093/oxfordhb/9780199639755.013.5

Saavedra, M. J. (2016). *Eldercare 101: A practical guide to later life planning, care, and Well-being*. Rowman & Littlefield.

Sandwich generation: Strike a better life balance with these tips. (2023). Amy's Helping Hands. https://www.amyshelpinghands.ca/caregiver-support-74/sandwich-generation-strike-a-better-life-balance-with-these-tips

Saran, C. (2023, September 2). *Helpful daily activities for dementia patients: 50 expert tips and suggestions to keep your loved one engaged.* English. https://www.pgs-nhcare.com/helpful-daily-activities-for-dementia-patients-50-expert-tips-and-suggestions-to-keep-your-loved-one-engaged

Seladi-Schulman, J. (2020, May 13). *What does medicare cover if you have dementia?* Healthline. https://www.healthline.com/health/medicare/does-medicare-cover-dementia-care

Segal, J., Smith, M., Robinson, L., & Boose, G. (2023, November 7). *Nonverbal communication and body language*. HelpGuide.org. https://www.helpguide.org/articles/relationships-communication/nonverbal-communication.htm

Sestito, N., Bodenheimer, L., & White, C. P. (2019). What Primary Care Physicians Need To Know About Dementia. *MD Advisor: A Journal for New Jersey Medical Community, 12*(3), 9–15.

Stephan, A., Möhler, R., Renom-Guiteras, A., & Meyer, G. (2015). Successful collaboration in dementia care from the perspectives of healthcare professionals and informal carers in Germany: Results from a focus group study. *BMC Health Services Research, 15*(1). https://doi.org/10.1186/s12913-015-0875-3

Sutcliffe, D. (2004). *Introducing dementia: The essential facts and issues of care*. Age Concern England.

The compound effect summary. (2021, August 5). What You Will Learn. https://www.whatyouwilllearn.com/book/the-compound-effect/

There is no failure, only feedback (2021). drcherrycoaching.com. https://drcherrycoaching.com/wp-content/uploads/2021/02/There-Is-No-Failure-Only-Feedback-.pdf

Tori, K., Kalligeros, M., Nanda, A., Shehadeh, F., van Aalst, R., Chit, A., & Mylonakis, E. (2020, July 31). Association between dementia and psychiatric disorders in long-term care residents. *Medicine, 99*(31). https://doi.org/10.1097/md.0000000000021412

Types of dementia. (2023). Alzheimer's Disease International (ADI). https://www.alzint.org/about/dementia-facts-figures/types-of-dementia

VanBooven, V. (2007, October 9). *The working caregiver: Issues faced with caregiving while employed.* AgingCare.com. https://www.agingcare.com/Articles/Caregiving-Issues-and-work-95637.htm

Vock, J. (2021, January 15). *Helping someone with dementia who has apraxia.* Elizz. https://www.elizz.com/caregiver-resources/dementia-care/helping-someone-with-dementia-who-has-apraxia/

Weatherill, G. (2020). *The caregiver's guide to dementia: Practical advice for caring for yourself and your loved one.* Rockridge Press.

What is geriatric psychiatry and how can it help my loved one? (2022, June 15). The Kensington Reston. https://kensingtonreston.com/geriatric-psychiatry/

Why nutrition is important for people with dementia. (2020, October). Social Care Institute for Excellence. https://www.scie.org.uk/dementia/living-with-dementia/eating-well/importance-of-nutrition.asp

Willis, E., Semple, A. C., & de Waal, H. (2016). Quantifying the benefits of peer support for people with dementia: A social return on investment (SROI) study. *Dementia, 17*(3), 266–278. https://doi.org/10.1177/1471301216640184

Wong, W. (2020, August 17). Economic burden of alzheimer disease and managed care considerations. *The American Journal of Managed Care, 26*(Suppl 8). https://doi.org/10.37765/ajmc.2020.88482

World Health Organization. (2023, March 15). *Dementia.* World Health Organization. https://www.who.int/news-room/fact-sheets/detail/dementia

World Health Organization. (2021b, September 2). *World failing to address dementia challenge.* World Health Organization. https://www.who.int/news/item/02-09-2021-world-failing-to-address-dementia-challenge

World Health Organization. (2021a). *Towards a dementia-inclusive society: WHO toolkit for dementia-friendly initiatives (DFIs).* World Health Organization. https://iris.who.int/handle/10665/343780

Yu, D. S. F., Cheng, S.-T., & Wang, J. (2018). Unravelling positive aspects of caregiving in dementia: An integrative review of research literature. *International Journal of Nursing Studies, 79*, 1–26. https://doi.org/10.1016/j.ijnurstu.2017.10.008

APPENDIX : ADDITIONAL PROFESSIONS FOR YOUR DREAM TEAM

1. MEDICAL SPECIALISTS

PSYCHIATRIST

A psychiatrist is a doctor with expertise in understanding, treating, and preventing mental and emotional challenges. They use various medical, psychological, and social methods to assist individuals in coping with their symptoms and enhancing their mental well-being. General psychiatrists, while not specifically trained in geriatric psychiatry, are qualified to assess and treat mental health conditions, including those related to dementia. About two-thirds of people with dementia have at least one psychiatric diagnosis– with anxiety, depression, and insomnia being the most prevalent.

General psychiatrists can also provide assessment and treatment for family caregivers like you; who, in the challenging task of caring for a loved one with dementia, may experience significant strain. Managing the care of someone who requires constant attention can complicate family dynamics. And caregivers facing such challenges may indeed encounter psychiatric conditions. If you suspect mental health concerns for yourself or your loved one (such as anxiety or depression), consider meeting with a psychiatrist.

To find a psychiatrist, visit https://finder.psychiatry.org/, or seek a referral from your general practitioner. Medicare may cover assessments or depression screenings, but only for psychiatrists who participate in Medicare. You can choose this as a search criterion in the American Psychiatric Association search tool (available at: finder.psychiatry.org).

In your session(s) with a psychiatrist, you might want to ask questions like:

- Can my loved one be assessed for anxiety and depression?
- What kind of medication is prescribed for these symptoms?
- Can hallucinations, agitation, irritability, psychosis, insomnia, or disinhibition (whatever your loved one's symptoms are) be managed with medication?
- Which medications should we look into, and what are the possible adverse effects?

How to partner with a psychiatrist

Be very factual in describing the behavior of your loved one with dementia. Portray your loved one's observable behaviors and your interpretation of them. Be upfront if *you* need help, but do not use your loved one's sessions to cover your own depression.

NEUROPSYCHOLOGIST

A neuropsychologist is a psychologist who specializes in neurological brain disorders and behaviors resulting from those disorders. They generally assess their patients' cognitive abilities through computerized tests. Their primary focus is research, although they may offer therapy services. They are often involved in atypical dementia evaluation.

When and where to find a neuropsychologist?

As soon as your loved one starts developing the first symptoms of dementia, it may be a good time to get a neuropsychological evaluation. To find a board-certified neuropsychologist in your area, use the AACN search engine at https://theaacn.org/directory/.

Medicare may cover neuropsychological evaluations and tests if they are deemed medically necessary. For information about Medicare coverage relative to neuropsychological testing, visit www.cms.gov and type "Psychological and Neuropsychological Testing" in the website's search engine.

What to ask a neuropsychologist?

Here are a few questions you might want to ask a neuropsychologist when you meet them for the first time:

- What kind of test is my loved one going to take?
- Do these tests lead to a precise dementia diagnosis?
- What is the purpose of each test?
- Will these evaluations determine how advanced the dementia is?
- What can my expectations for my loved one with dementia be?
- How can I help my loved one maintain cognitive health for as long as possible?

How to partner with a neuropsychologist?

Make sure your loved one takes all the tests recommended by the neuropsychologist. These healthcare professionals are experts in their field, so follow their guidance.

2. CARE AND SUPPORT PROFESSIONALS

PHYSIOTHERAPIST/PHYSICAL THERAPIST

Physical therapists (physiotherapists) are healthcare professionals focusing on treating physical disabilities and impairments. They assist individuals in recovering from injuries, managing chronic diseases, and enhancing mobility, function, and quality of life. They use physical treatments like exercise, massage, and manipulation to reach these goals.

A physiotherapist assesses and works with your loved one (and you) to design exercise programs that can slow down or alleviate the progression of dementia symptoms. While physiotherapists primarily address physical needs, they may also attend to emotional, cognitive, and social issues.

Physical therapists also work preventatively to decrease the probability of developing dementia, as conditions such as high blood pressure, diabetes, and brain injuries are correlated with dementia. Although dementia cannot be cured or stopped, its associated symptoms can be tempered. Physiotherapy can delay the onset of dementia by slowing down the progression of symptoms, such as the incapacity to perform activities of daily living or tasks that involve cognitive thinking.

When to consult a physiotherapist?

Visiting a physical therapist is highly recommended as soon as you notice the first signs of cognitive decline in your loved one.

Original Medicare Part B generally covers physical therapy for an annually capped amount. For more information on the current cap, refer to the American Physical Therapy Association's website. Type "Medicare payment thresholds for outpatient therapy services" in the search bar, and look at the "PT" (physical therapy) amount for the current year.

What to ask a physiotherapist?

Here are a few questions you might want to ask the physiotherapist before your loved one starts their sessions:

- What is your philosophy and therapy approach?
- What kind of exercises do you recommend for preventing falls?
- What do you need to know about my loved one with dementia to provide better care?
- How do you handle situations where a patient with dementia refuses to cooperate?
- Can you please provide proof of your accreditation and continuing education credits?

Where to find a physiotherapist?

When you want to employ the services of a physiotherapist, you can use the tools provided below to find one:

https://www.choosept.com/guide/physical-therapy-guide-alzheimers-disease

https://aptaapps.apta.org//APTAPTDirectory/FindAPTDirectory.aspx or type "apta find a physical therapist" in Google.

Whatever channel you use to find a physiotherapist, ensure they have the proper education and experience working specifically with dementia patients.

How to partner with a physiotherapist?

Collaborate with the physical therapist by sharing information about your loved one with dementia's preferences and habits at home. Discuss their gait and autonomy, and report your observations as much as possible in a factual and unbiased way. Work together to help them help you.

SPEECH AND LANGUAGE THERAPIST

A speech and language therapist (SLT), or speech and language pathologist (SLP) or just speech therapist, is a healthcare professional specializing in diagnosing, treating, and caring for individuals of all ages who face communication disorders. These disorders may present themselves as challenges in speech, language, fluency, literacy, voice, or physical difficulties related to eating or swallowing.

Speech and language pathologists offer assistance and techniques to individuals in the early stages of dementia who experience speech problems. They aim to help individuals refine their communication abilities for more precise and effective speech. They may also play a role in diagnosing certain types of dementia that impact language, such as Primary Progressive Aphasia, the second major form of frontotemporal dementia.

A speech and language therapist does the following:

- Assesses difficulties with swallowing (dysphagia) and communication (speech and comprehension).

- Provides treatment recommendations based on the assessment.
- Offers speech and articulation exercises.
- Provides attention, memory, problem-solving, and higher-level thinking exercises.
- Assists with food choices and nutrition when swallowing becomes challenging.
- Supports caregivers in effectively communicating with their loved ones with dementia, and assists with speech exercises.
- In the latter stages of dementia, where eating and swallowing issues may emerge, a speech and language pathologist can advise on the safest approach to offer food and water to your loved one.

When to consult a speech and language therapist?

You and your loved one should visit a speech and language therapist when:

- Communication (speech or comprehension) becomes difficult for your loved one with dementia.
- Your loved one with dementia starts experiencing difficulties with eating, drinking, or swallowing.

What to ask a speech and language therapist?

Here are a few questions you might want to ask a speech and language therapist:

- What can I expect from this treatment?
- How much experience do you have in dementia care?
- How long will it take for a complete and comprehensive evaluation?
- What are the common mistakes to avoid during my loved one's mealtime?

Where to find a speech and language therapist?

To find a speech and language therapist, you can use the search tool on the American Speech-Language-Hearing Association website. You can also seek referrals from your loved one's primary care physician or other healthcare providers. Note that you may not have to leave the comfort of your home to consult an SLT, as many speech and language therapists propose "telehealth" services in addition to their regular consultations.

Medicare Part B covers outpatient speech and language pathology services as long as they are deemed medically necessary. You may obtain a refund of up to 80% of the Medicare-approved amount. In addition to the Part-B deductible, 20% will be at your charge. Medicaid also covers speech and language pathology services for people with dementia, but coverage varies depending on the state.

How to partner with a speech and language therapist?

Ask questions about dementia. Also, ask questions about specific problems you have encountered with your loved one with dementia. Collaborate to the best of your ability to implement the strategies that the speech and language pathologist recommends. Do not hesitate to mention all the emotions you are going through when using one of the strategies they recommended.

LICENSED MARRIAGE AND FAMILY THERAPIST

Marriage and Family Therapists (MFTs) help families navigate the challenges of caring for a loved one with dementia by addressing communication challenges, resolving conflicts related to caregiving decisions, and providing support through ambiguous loss and the evolving stages of dementia. Additionally, MFTs offer comfort to families during the final days of their loved one's life.

When and Where to Consult a Marriage and Family Therapist?

Consider consulting an MFT if you encounter challenges in solving family disagreements, seek increased social support, need guidance to help your loved one maximize their potential, or desire more balance in the family.

To find an MFT, visit www.therapistlocator.net or the "find a therapist" tab on the American Family Therapy Academy website (www.afta.org).

Federal Law Update Regarding Medicare/Medicaid:

In 2023, Congress passed an historic federal law allowing Medicare Part B coverage for Marriage and Family Therapy (MFT) and Mental Health Counseling (MHC) services. Effective January 1st, 2024, MFTs can serve Medicare enrollees and receive reimbursements. For more information, visit the "Advance the Profession" section on the AAMFT website. What to ask during your first meeting with an MFT:

- How do you help families navigate conflicts related to caregiving decisions, finances, and legal matters related to dementia care?
- What is your approach to providing comfort and support throughout the progression of dementia?
- How can your approach help our family face the unique challenges related to dementia care?
- Do you offer sliding scale fees for your services?

How to Partner with a Marriage and Family Therapist?

Be open and honest during sessions. MFTs are there to help, not to judge. Set clear goals and objectives, and take action based on the discussions that take place during therapy sessions.

RECREATIONAL THERAPISTS / DIVERSIONAL THERAPISTS

Recreational therapists use leisure activities to improve well-being in the physical, emotional, and cognitive domains. To maximize the enjoyment, engagement, and well-being of your loved one with dementia, recreational therapists design activities such as music, art, crafts, reading, reminiscence, pets, etc., based on your loved one's preferences. Recreational therapists also involve individuals with dementia and their caregivers in customizing a unique activity plan. Most of the time, recreational therapists are employees of residential aged-care institutions and aged-care units, but they may also work for community programs to assist socially isolated individuals at home.

When to hire a recreational therapist?

It wouldn't hurt to consult a recreational therapist as soon as your loved one receives a dementia diagnosis. Then, the recreational therapist can work with them through all the stages to slow down the progression of dementia symptoms for as long as possible. Their services are especially pertinent if your loved one is socially isolated, agitated, or aggressive.

What to ask a certified therapeutic recreation specialist?

When hiring a recreational therapist for your loved one, ask them about their experience working with individuals with dementia, their certifications and qualifications, and the recreational activities they typically use. Also, ask them how you can contribute to your loved one's activity plan. Recreational therapists should have no trouble designing one that involves you.

Where to find a certified therapeutic recreation specialist?

It is safer to use the services of certified professionals, as those generally follow a code of ethics. To find a certified therapeutic recreational specialist (CTRS), use the "CTRS verification" tab on the National Council for Therapeutic Recreation Certification's website. Additionally, many healthcare facilities, such as hospitals and long-term care facilities, may employ certified recreational therapists. Finally, you may ask your loved one's social worker for referrals to accredited recreational therapists in your area.

Medicare and Medicaid do not currently cover certified therapeutic recreation specialists' services, except when offered in multidisciplinary rehabilitation programs. However, some private insurance plans do. Verify directly with your loved one's insurance provider.

How to partner with a certified therapeutic recreation specialist?

Collaborate with your loved one's recreational therapist to develop your loved one's personalized activity plan. Treat your loved one's recreational therapist as an expert in their field. Consider their role as crucial as other healthcare professionals' roles, and regularly communicate with them about the effectiveness that the personalized activity plan is having on your loved one's behaviors.

ART THERAPIST

Art therapists utilize the power of art to delve into feelings, emotions, memories, and behaviors, uncovering unspoken symbols in the process. Through expressive art, and storytelling, art therapists enhance the quality of life for your loved one with dementia and yourself.

Art therapy is particularly beneficial during the mild and moderate phases of dementia. You can locate a board-certified art therapist in the United States through the Art Therapy Credentials Board (ATCB)'s website at https://www.atcb.org by typing "find a credentialed art therapist" in the search bar. If you're in Canada, visit https://www.canadianarttherapy.org, click on the "find an art therapist" tab, and select "search the directory."

When meeting with an art therapist, kickstart the conversation with questions like:

- How can art therapy benefit my loved one?
- In what ways can art therapy help my loved one with dementia process emotions and navigate psychological challenges?
- What training or credentials have you received in art therapy?
- Can you share insights into your approach to art therapy?
- Could you provide examples of successful outcomes from your practice?

Like in music therapy, whether you are seeking art therapy for yourself, your loved one with dementia, or joint sessions involving both, ensure that your clinical goals are explicitly communicated during the referral or self-referral process.

DANCE-MOVEMENT THERAPISTS

In their general clinical practice, Dance-movement therapists use dance and movement to observe, assess, and realize treatment plans for their clients to:

- Improve body image and self-esteem
- Develop effective communication skills
- Expand their movement vocabulary
- Gain insight into patterns of behavior
- Create new options for coping with problems.

In their general clinical practice, dance therapists conduct research and collaborate with multidisciplinary teams of healthcare professionals, documenting their work in clinical records. In dementia care, dance therapists focus on keeping clients active, as exercise has been shown to slow down the progression of dementia symptoms.

Beyond the physical benefits, dance-movement therapy is also a powerful tool for emotional well-being. In dance-movement therapy, individuals with dementia engage in movement that provides a unique channel for self-expression, connection with emotions, and moments of joy. Simultaneously, caregivers can find emotional support and regulation, making it a valuable respite activity that contributes to their own mental health. Overall, the expressive and creative nature of movement allows for a shared emotional experience, fostering a sense of connection and well-being for individuals with dementia and their caregivers.

When and where to consult a dance movement therapist?

You can consult a dance-movement therapist for as long as your loved one with dementia can move safely. Dance-movement therapy may be adapted in mild, moderate, and even part of the severe stages of dementia, given that most physical impairments tend to appear in the last stage of dementia.

To find a certified dance-movement therapist in the United States, search the American Dance Therapy Association (ADTA) website at https://www.adta.org/find-a-dmt#/ and filter using the term "dementia".

Here are a few questions you may want to ask the dance-movement therapist when you start your sessions:

- How is dance-movement therapy different from regular dancing?
- Do you have experience in dance therapy with older adults with dementia?
- How do you mitigate the risk of falls in dance-movement therapy sessions?
- Do you actively keep up-to-date in your clinical practice through continuing education?

How to partner with a dance-movement therapist

Provide referral information such as the family history of your loved one with dementia, skills, movement limitations, strengths, current stage, and evolution of the condition. List symptoms, limitations, and provide information about medication that may hinder movement.

DRAMA THERAPIST

Drama therapists use drama as a therapeutic approach and creative form of expression to assist individuals in improving their emotional well-being. In the context of dementia care, drama therapists generally target goals in similar domains to music therapists: in the emotional area, they may, for example, aim to address depressive symptoms or encourage expression and self-regulation through guided improvisation. In the cognitive domain, they may seek to improve attention, or stimulate memory and problem-solving skills through storytelling, role-playing, and improvisation. In the social area, their goal might be strengthening the bond between your loved one with dementia and yourself, their caregiver, through collaborative activities such as shared storytelling, promoting communication, and joint experiences.

When and where to consult a drama therapist?

Consulting a drama therapist is most beneficial in the mild to moderate stages, when your loved one with dementia retains sufficient cognitive and emotional engagement to participate meaningfully in drama therapy. Yet, although less frequent, drama therapy can be used in the severe stage of dementia to address existential issues that are particularly relevant when nearing the end of life. To find a drama therapist who works in dementia care, use the search tool of the North American Drama Therapy Association (NADTA) website at https://www.nadta.org/find-a-drama-therapist#/ and filter using the "Alzheimer's/Dementia" keywords.

When you meet a drama therapist for the first time, here are a few questions you can ask:

- Can you tell me more about your experience in dementia care?
- What is your approach to drama therapy?
- Do you actively pursue continuing education in your practice?
- Are you an NADTA member?

How to partner with a drama therapist

Prioritize effective communication. Share relevant details about your loved one, express clear goals, and communicate your needs as a caregiver. Use therapy sessions as respite and trust the therapist's expertise. Maintain open communication, be receptive to feedback, and consider joint sessions to nurture a positive relationship with your loved one with dementia.

3. CARE COORDINATION AND LEGAL SUPPORT

GERIATRIC CARE MANAGER

Geriatric care managers specialize in offering support and resources to older adults and their families, often functioning similarly to social workers. Although typically trained as social workers, nurses, or gerontologists, these professionals operate in the private sector, thereby distinguishing them from social workers, who primarily work in the public sector with larger caseloads. In dementia care, geriatric care managers are crucial in coordinating and ensuring the well-being of your loved one and their environment.

When and where to find a geriatric care manager?

From the moment your loved one starts displaying behaviors that could be harmful, whether physically, socially, psychologically, or financially, such as forgetting to pay bills, forgetting to eat, or overeating, it is time to consider a geriatric care manager who will act like a professional extension of the family caregiver. You can find a geriatric care manager through organizations such as aarp.org, eldercare locator, caring.com, and Aging Life Care Association. You can also find a geriatric care manager by word of mouth in dementia caregiver support groups. When you meet a geriatric care manager for the first time, you can ask things like:

- Do you have experience in dementia care? Tell me more about it.
- What would you do to neutralize a crisis?
- How can you help relieve stress for me, my loved one with dementia, and my family?
- Do you have a geriatric care manager certification or professional license?
- Can you provide client references?
- What is your fee structure and cost estimate (after they proceed to do the assessment of your loved one's needs)?

Medicare, Medicaid, and most private insurance (including insurance for long-term care) do not cover private geriatric care management, which is the main difference from a social worker. The initial assessment can cost between $400 and $800. Some long-term care insurance may cover this initial cost. After the evaluation, a geriatric care manager costs between $75 and $250 per hour, depending on your location (state and area).

How to partner with a geriatric care manager?

Clearly describe your loved one's medical, health, psychological, and special care needs. Explain the level of support required to cover their needs. Expose your constraints as a dementia caregiver.

4. HOME SUPPORT

HOUSEKEEPING

A housekeeping service provider is a company or individual that offers professional cleaning and maintenance services for homes, apartments, and other residential properties. These service providers typically employ trained and experienced housekeepers who can perform various tasks, including vacuuming, dusting, washing dishes, doing laundry, and keeping the house organized.

Housekeeping service providers can benefit dementia caregivers who lack the time or energy to clean their or their loved ones' home. They can also help families with young children or elderly members who may struggle with housekeeping tasks.

When to hire a housekeeper?

If you are the only caregiver and your loved one with dementia cannot be left alone, if you are exhausted or simply wondering whether you need help, it is probably time to hire someone. When choosing a housekeeping service provider, it's essential to consider factors such as the experience and reliability of the provider, the cost of their services, and their availability. Choosing a provider that has a good reputation for customer service is also important. An added bonus would be if they use environmentally-friendly cleaning products in their housekeeping tasks.

What to ask a housekeeper?

You should make sure to ask questions like the following:

- Do you have experience working with people with dementia?
- How long have you been working with older adults?

- Housekeeping providers can customize their services to meet each client's needs. For example, some service providers may offer weekly or bi-weekly cleaning services. In contrast, others may offer one-time deep cleaning services. The cost of these services varies depending on the frequency and scope of the cleaning, as well as the location and reputation of the service provider. Asking about schedule options would be a good idea.

Where to find a housekeeper?

If you want to hire a housekeeping service provider, your local Alzheimer's Association office or a social worker can help you get some references. Depending on the state, age, and level of autonomy of your loved one with dementia, Medicaid or Medicare may pay for housekeeping services.

How to partner with a housekeeper?

Give clear instructions, and have a task list ready. Your housekeeper may be able to help you with cleaning up the clutter in the house, and possibly even in adapting your home for physical safety (see Chapter 4). Initially, it might be difficult for your loved one with dementia to accept a stranger in the house, so it is advisable to stay present during the first few cleaning visits to reassure your loved one (and yourself) that it is safe. You can also use that time to demonstrate your preferred housekeeping methods.

MEAL DELIVERY SERVICES

These programs offer home-delivered meals to help provide well-balanced lunches and dinners. They also offer social interaction from the volunteers.

When to use meal delivery services?

If your loved one with dementia starts losing or gaining significant weight, and can no longer prepare or eat healthy meals autonomously, then it is time to use a meal delivery service.

Though primary Medicare does not cover meal delivery services, some Medicare "advantage plans" may include them.

QUICK REFERENCE GUIDE

Made in the USA
Las Vegas, NV
31 October 2026

56896240R00146